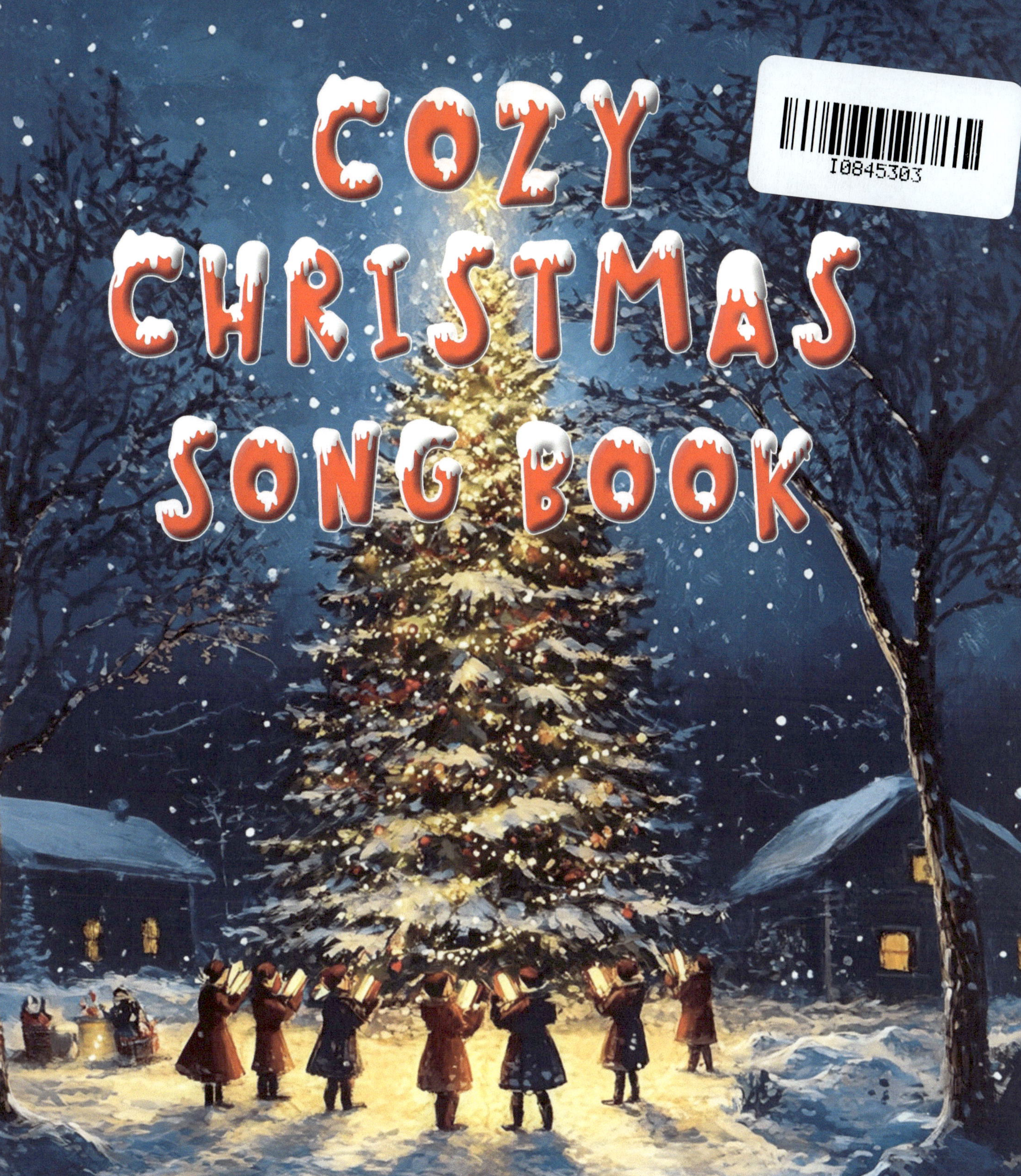
COZY CHRISTMAS SONG BOOK
© 2024 Comfy Corner Press
All Rights Reserved

JINGLE BELLS

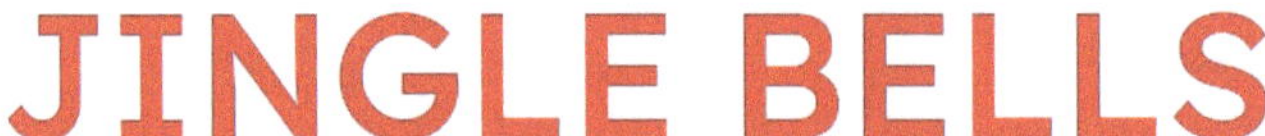

Jingle bells, jingle bells
Jingle all the way
Oh what fun it is to ride
In a one-horse open sleigh, O

Jingle bells, jingle bells
Jingle all the way
Oh what fun it is to ride
In a one-horse open sleigh.

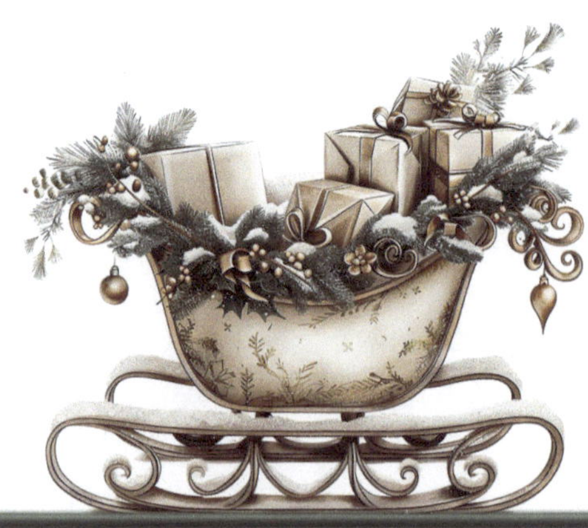

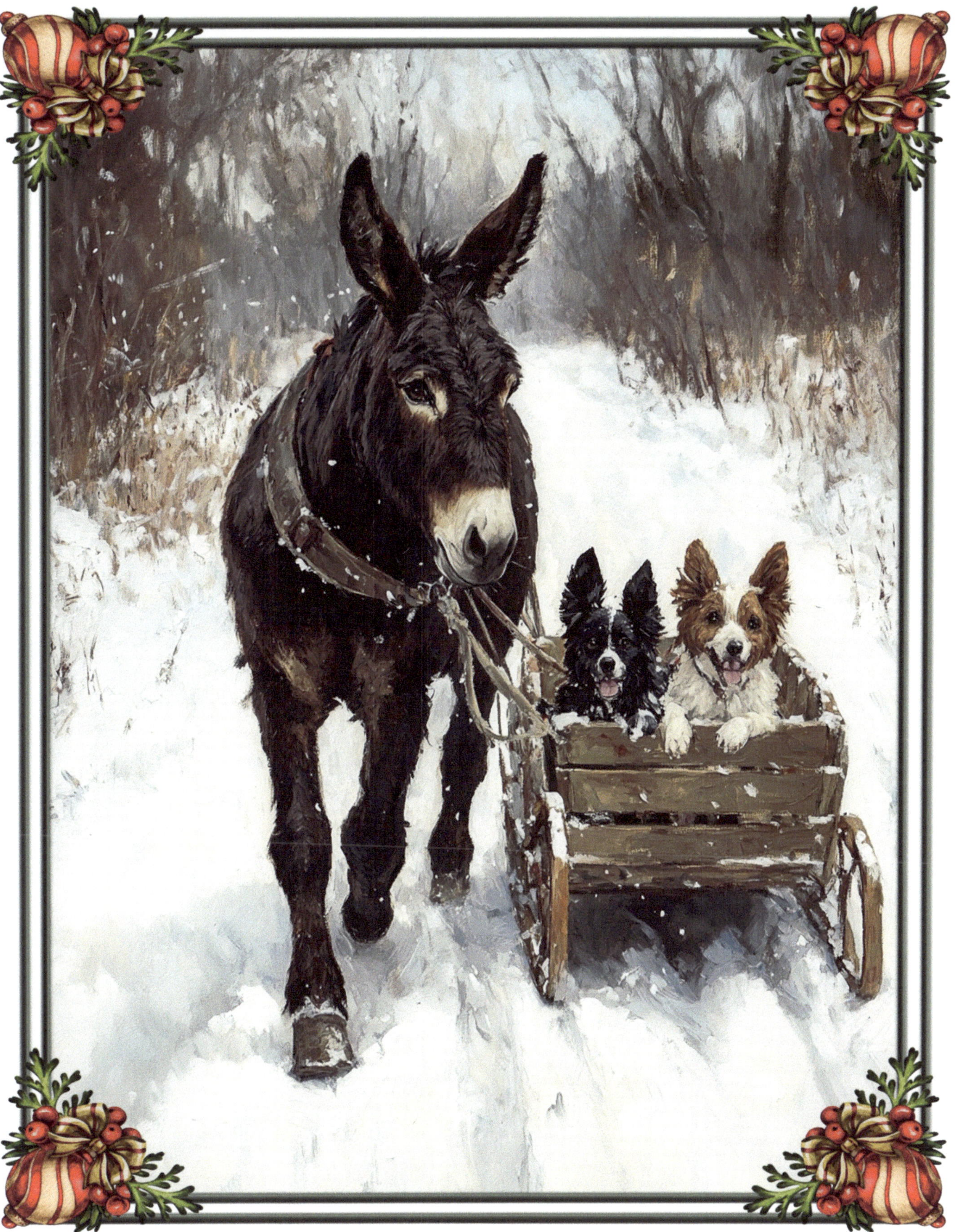

AWAY IN A MANGER

Away in a manger
No crib for a bed
The little Lord Jesus
Laid down His sweet head.

The stars in the bright sky
Looked down where He lay
The little Lord Jesus
Asleep on the hay.

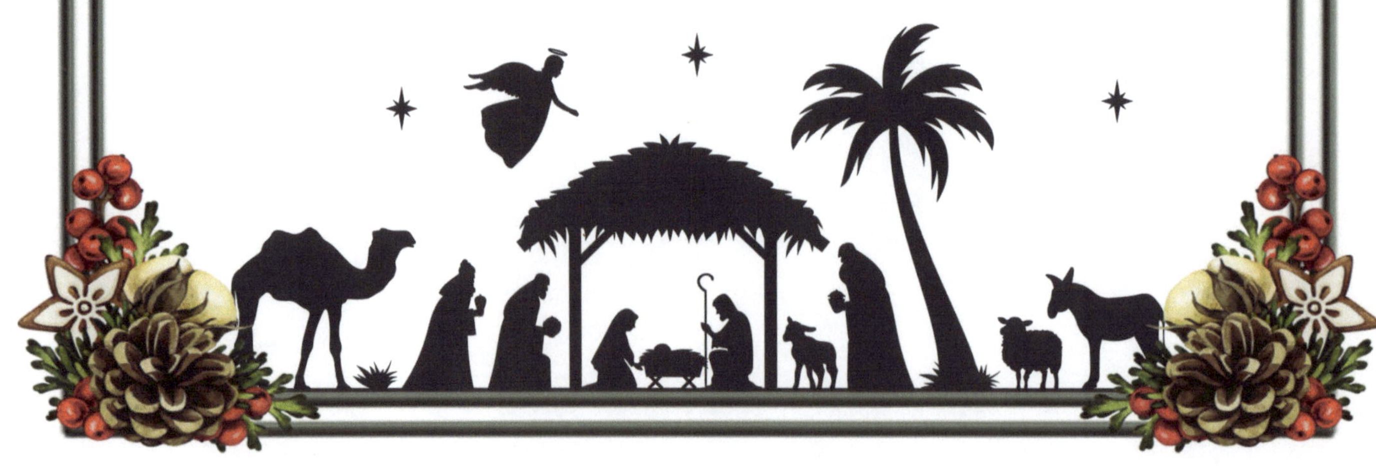

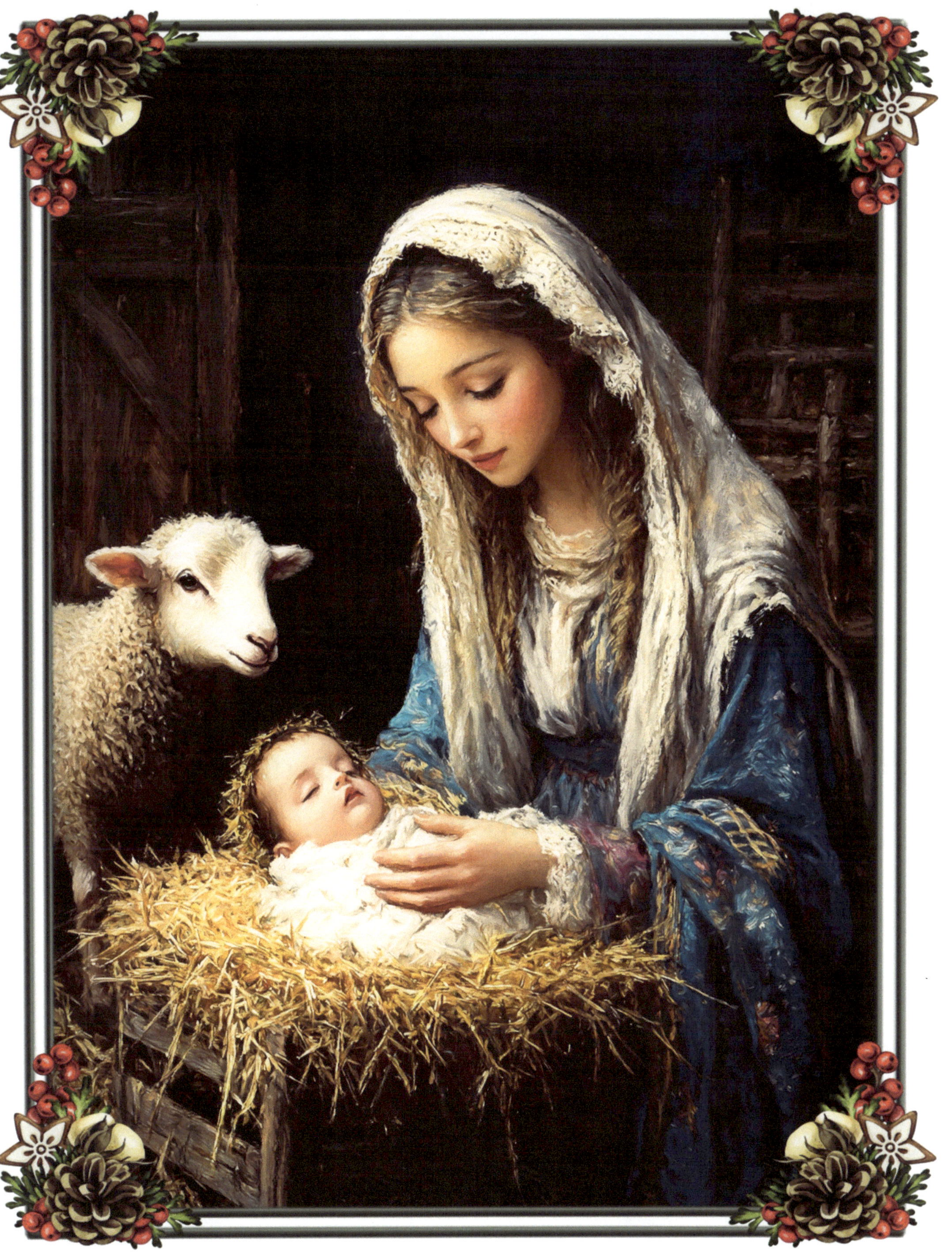

FROSTY THE SNOWMAN

Frosty the Snowman
was a jolly happy soul
With a corncob pipe
and a button nose
And two eyes made out of coal.

Frosty the Snowman
is a fairytale they say
He was made of snow
but the children know
That he came to life one day.

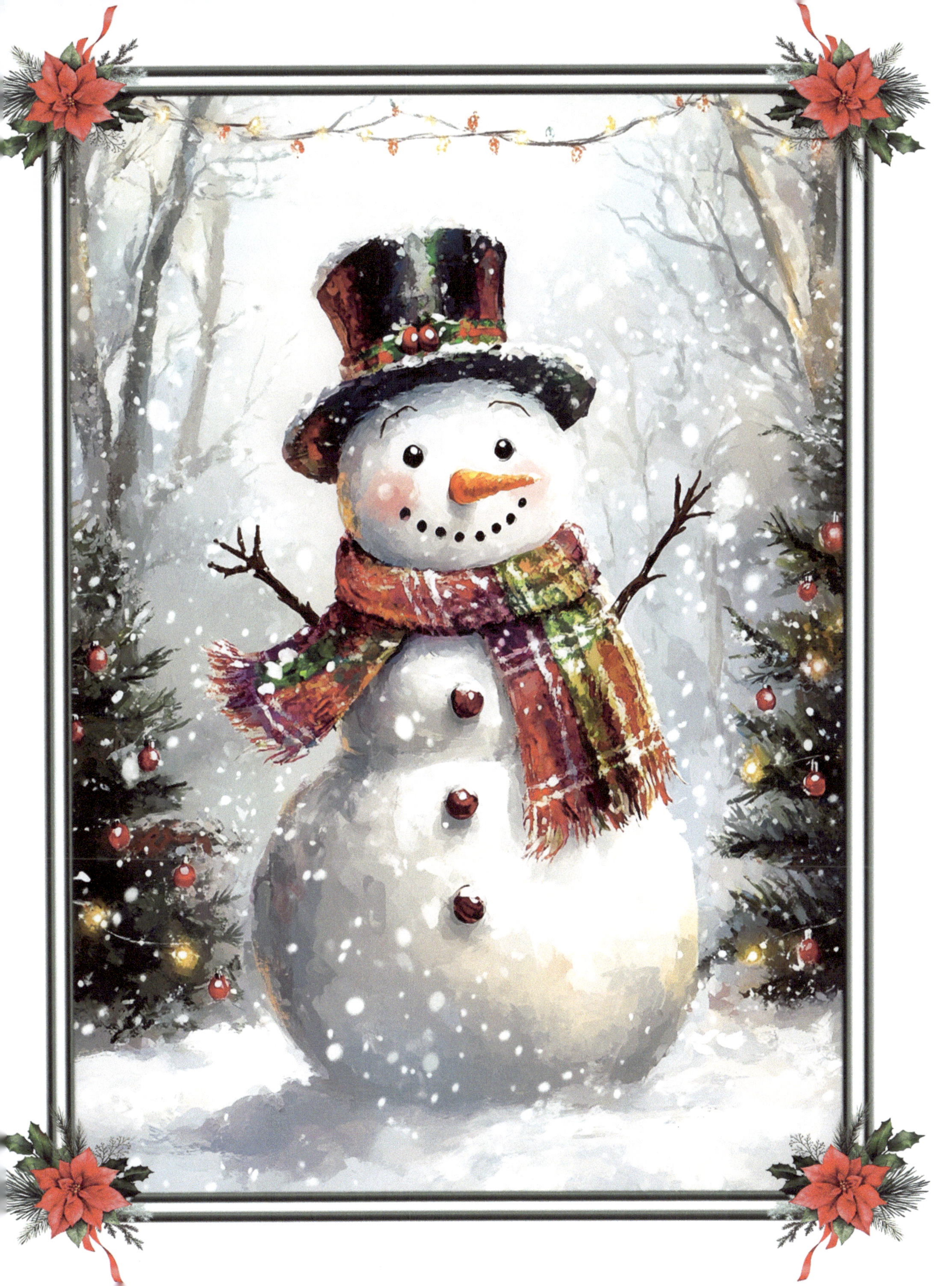

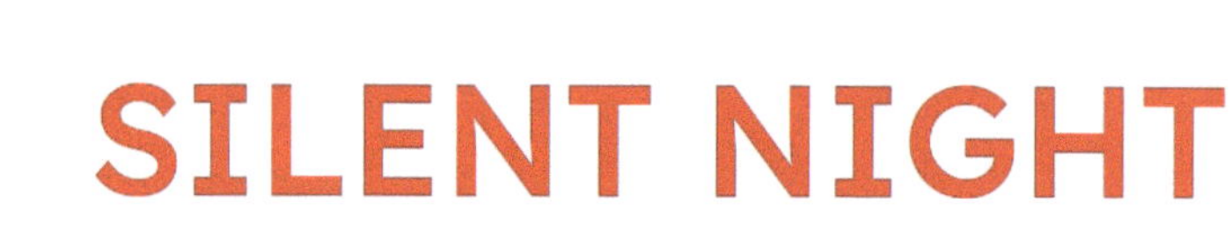

SILENT NIGHT

Silent night, Holy night
All is calm, all is bright.
Round yon Virgin
Mother and Child
Holy infant
So tender and mild

Sleep in Heavenly peace!
Sleep in Heavenly peace!

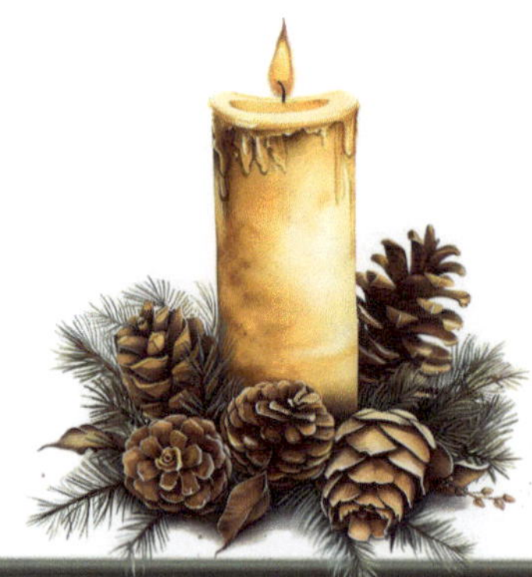

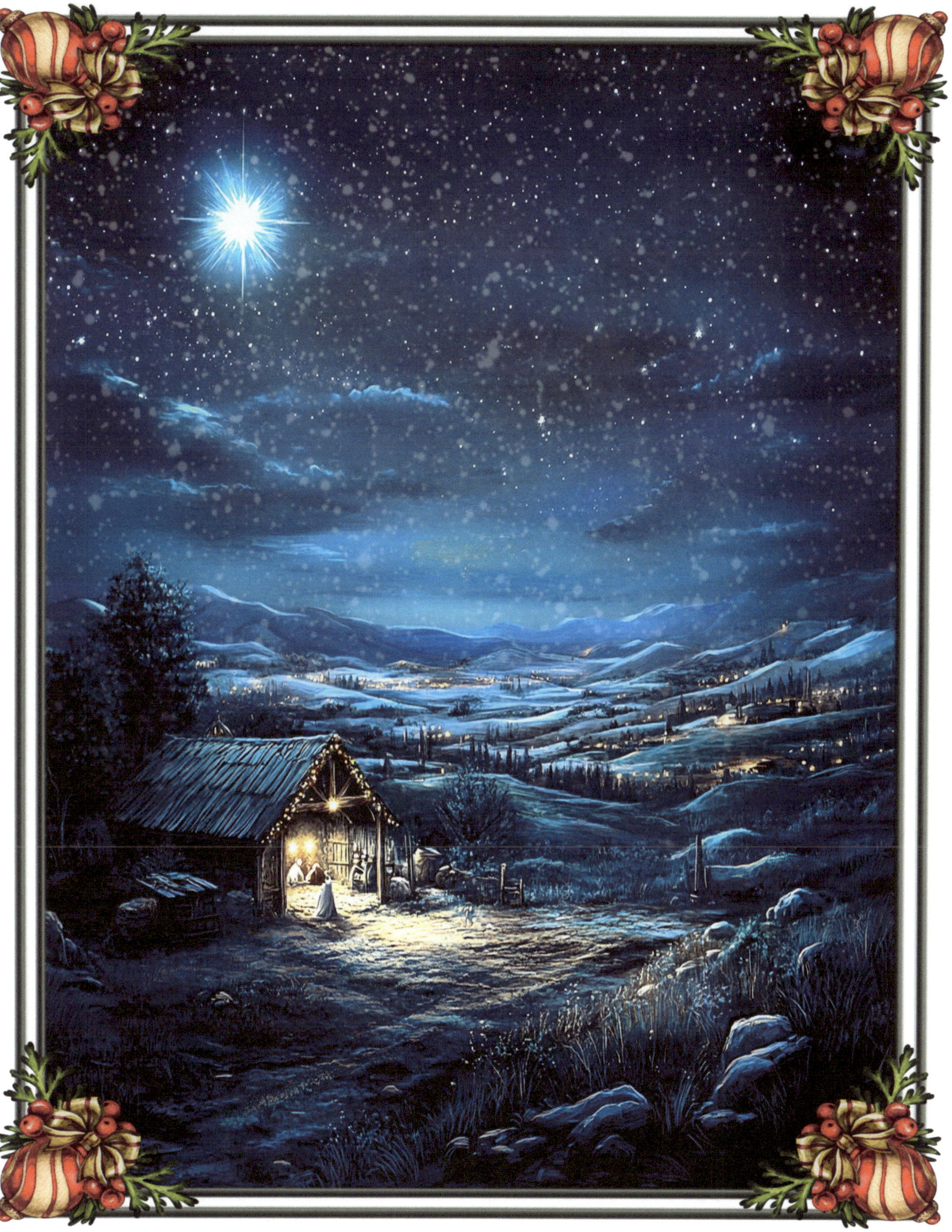

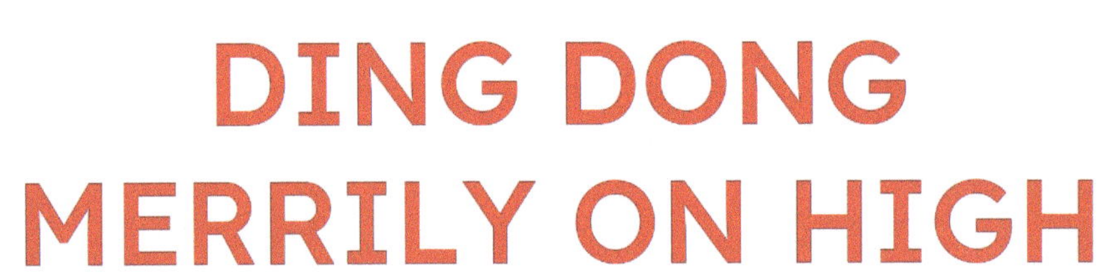

DING DONG MERRILY ON HIGH

Ding dong! merrily on high
In heav'n the bells are ringing.

Ding dong! verily the sky
Is riv'n with Angel singing.

Gloria,
Hosanna in excelsis!

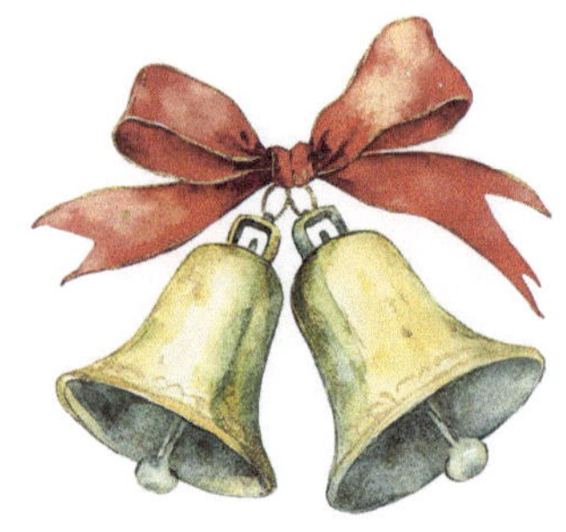

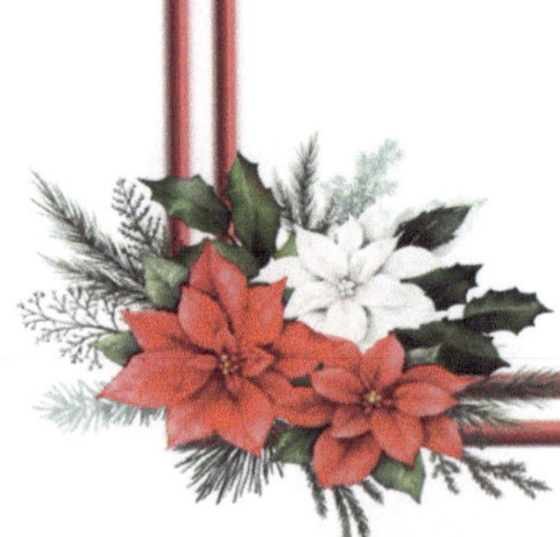

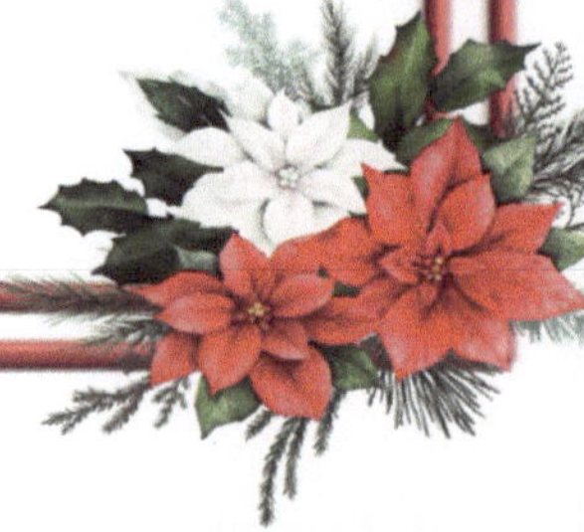

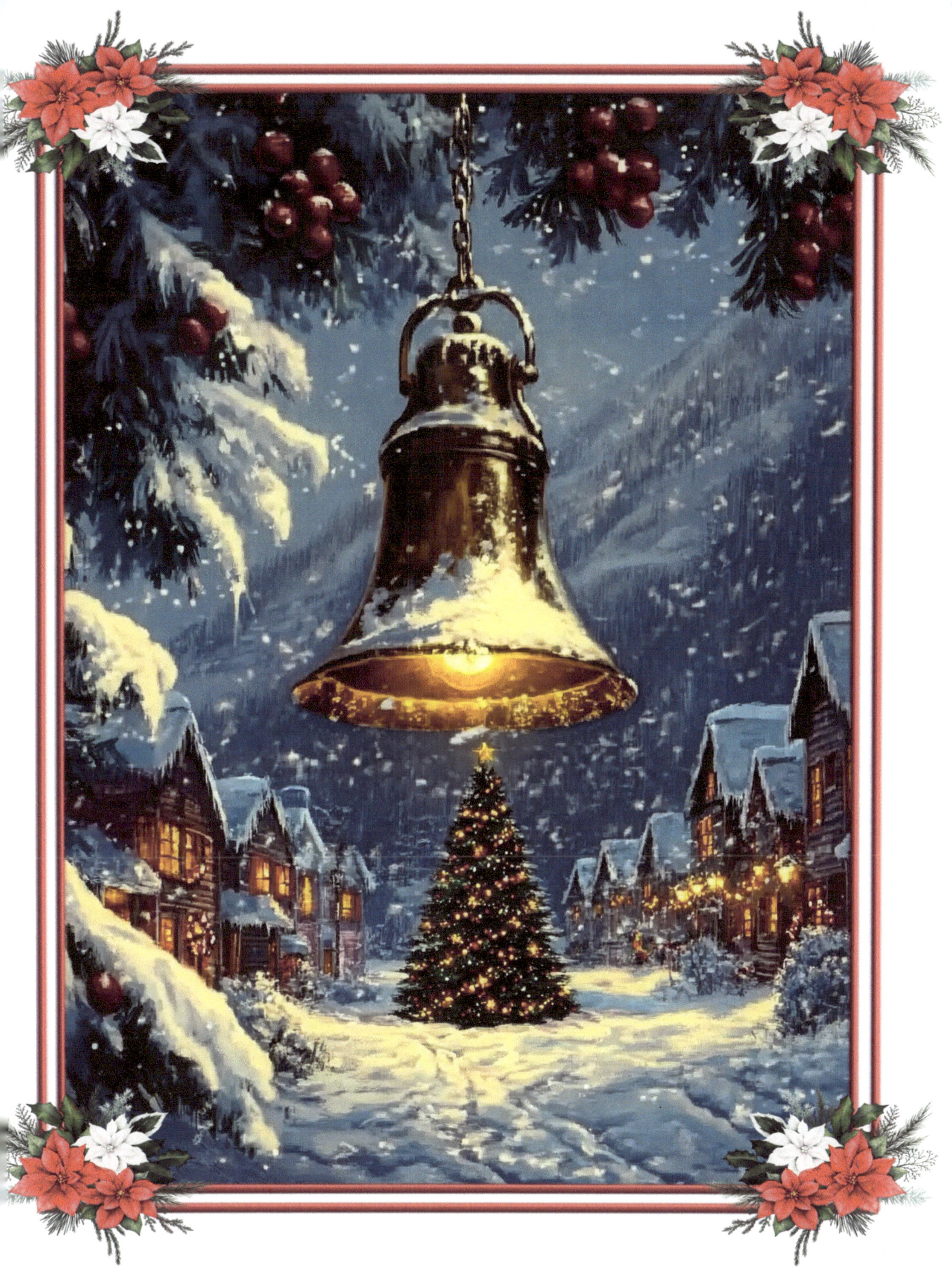

DECK THE HALLS

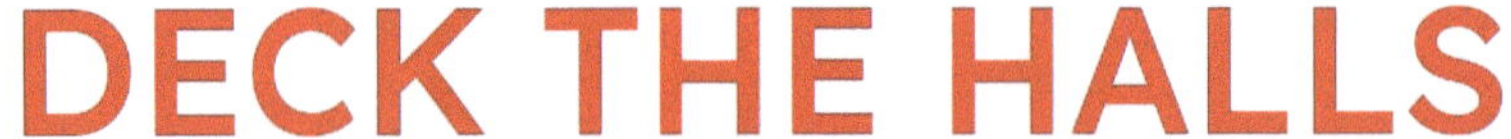

Deck the halls with
boughs of holly
Fa la la la la, la la la la.

'Tis the season to be jolly
Fa la la la la, la la la la.
Don we now our gay apparel
Fa la la, la la la, la la la.

Toll the ancient Yule tide carol
Fa la la la la, la la la la.

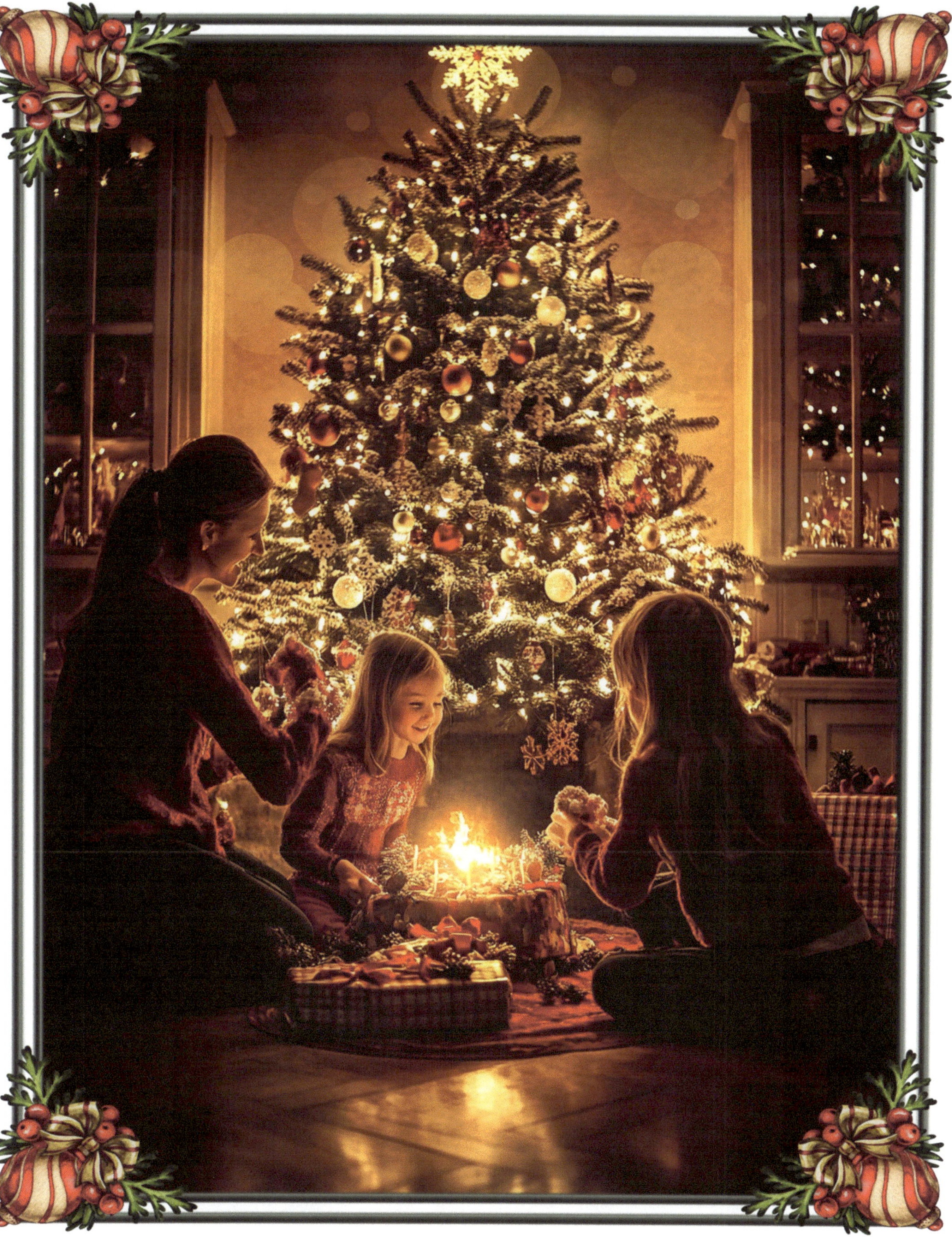

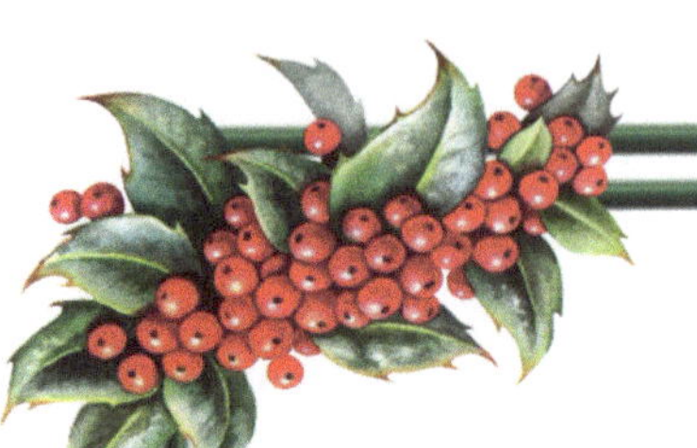 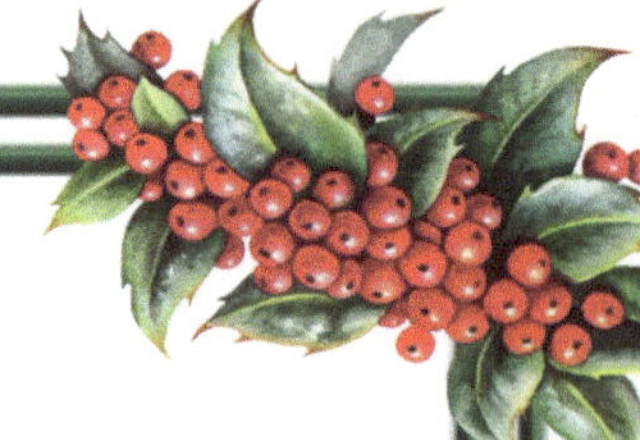

LET IT SNOW!

Oh the weather outside is frightful
but the fire is so delightful.

And since we've no place to go
Let It Snow! Let It Snow! Let It Snow!

It doesn't show signs of stopping
And I've brought some corn for popping.

The lights are turned way down low
Let It Snow! Let It Snow! Let It Snow!

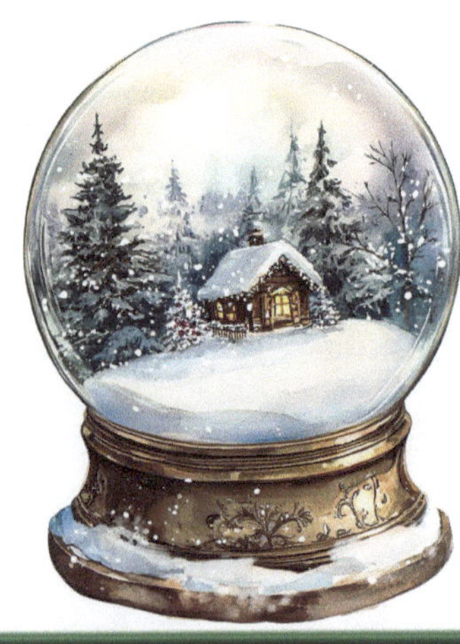

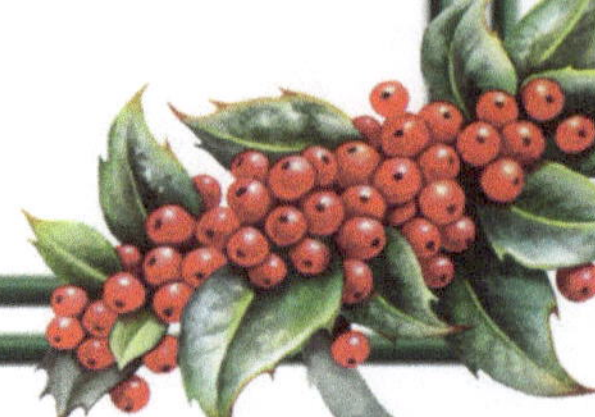

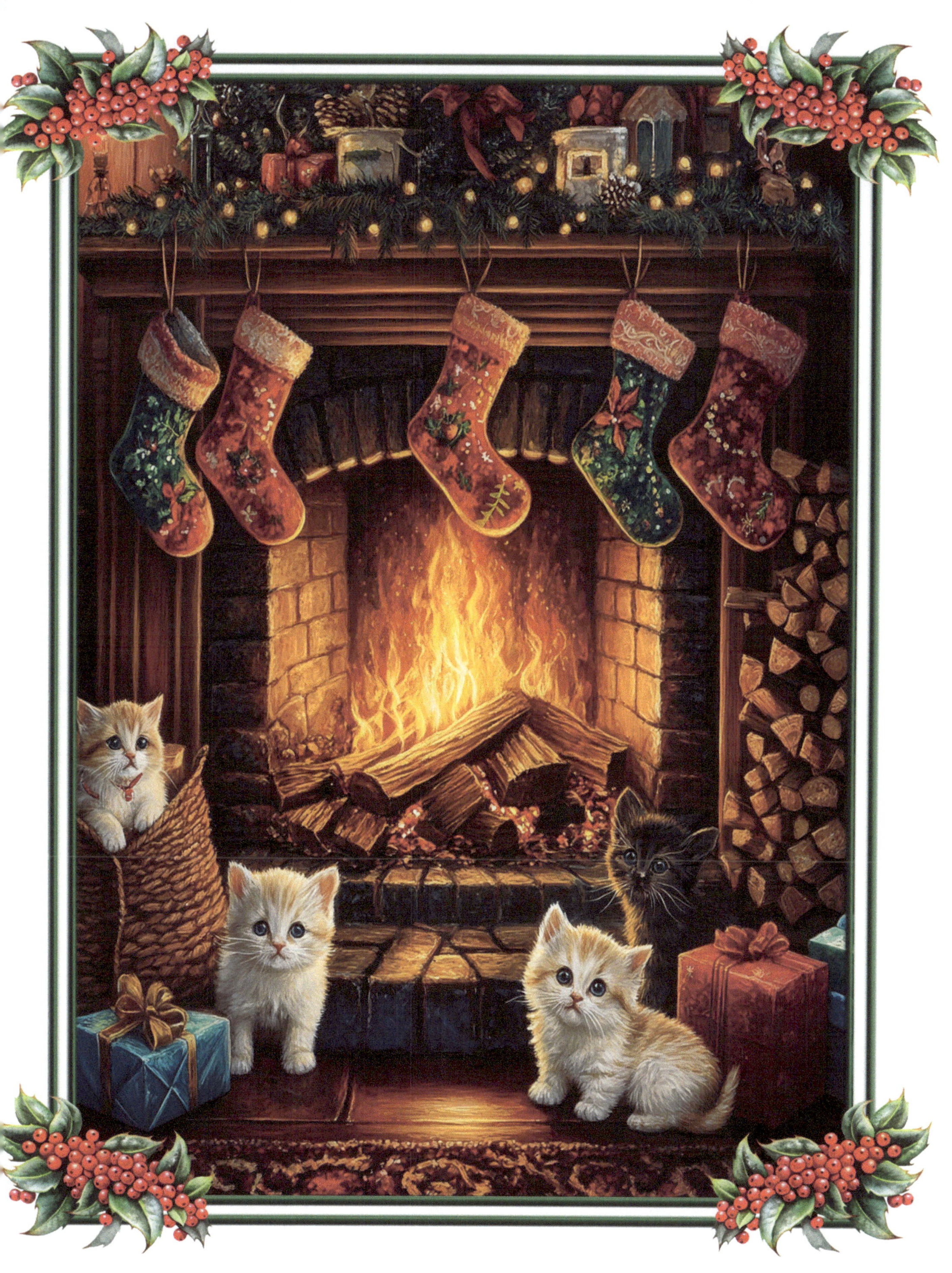

THE FIRST NOWELL

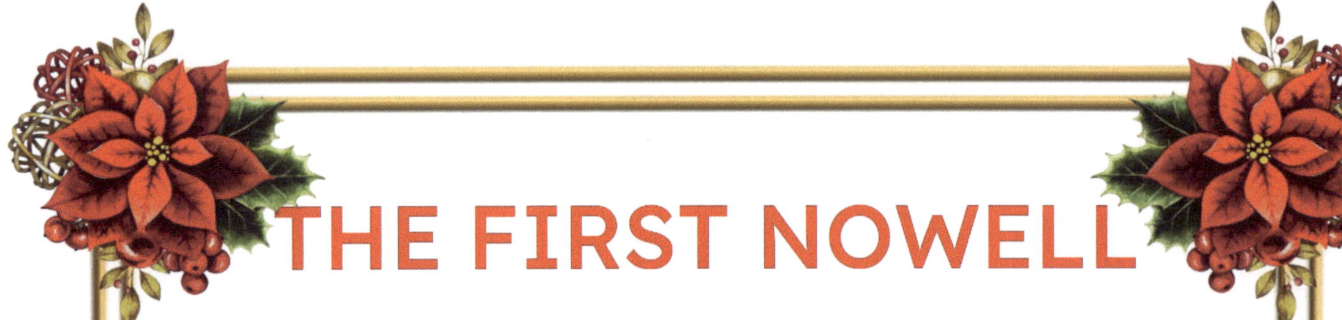

The first Nowell
the angels did say
Was to certain poor shepherds
in fields as they lay;

In fields where they
lay keeping their sheep,
On a cold winter's night
that was so deep.

Nowell! Nowell! Nowell! Nowell!
Born is the King of Israel!

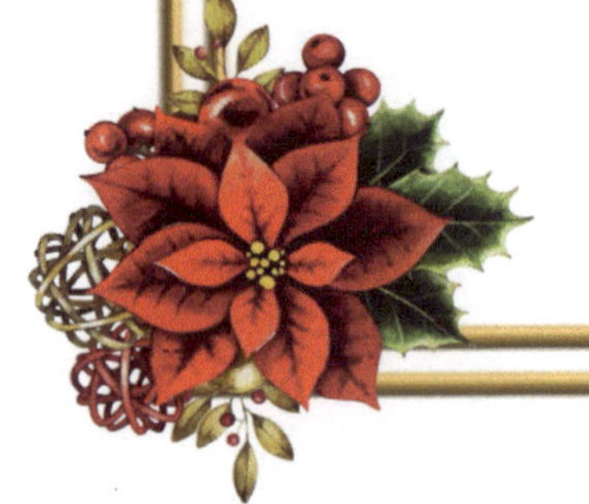

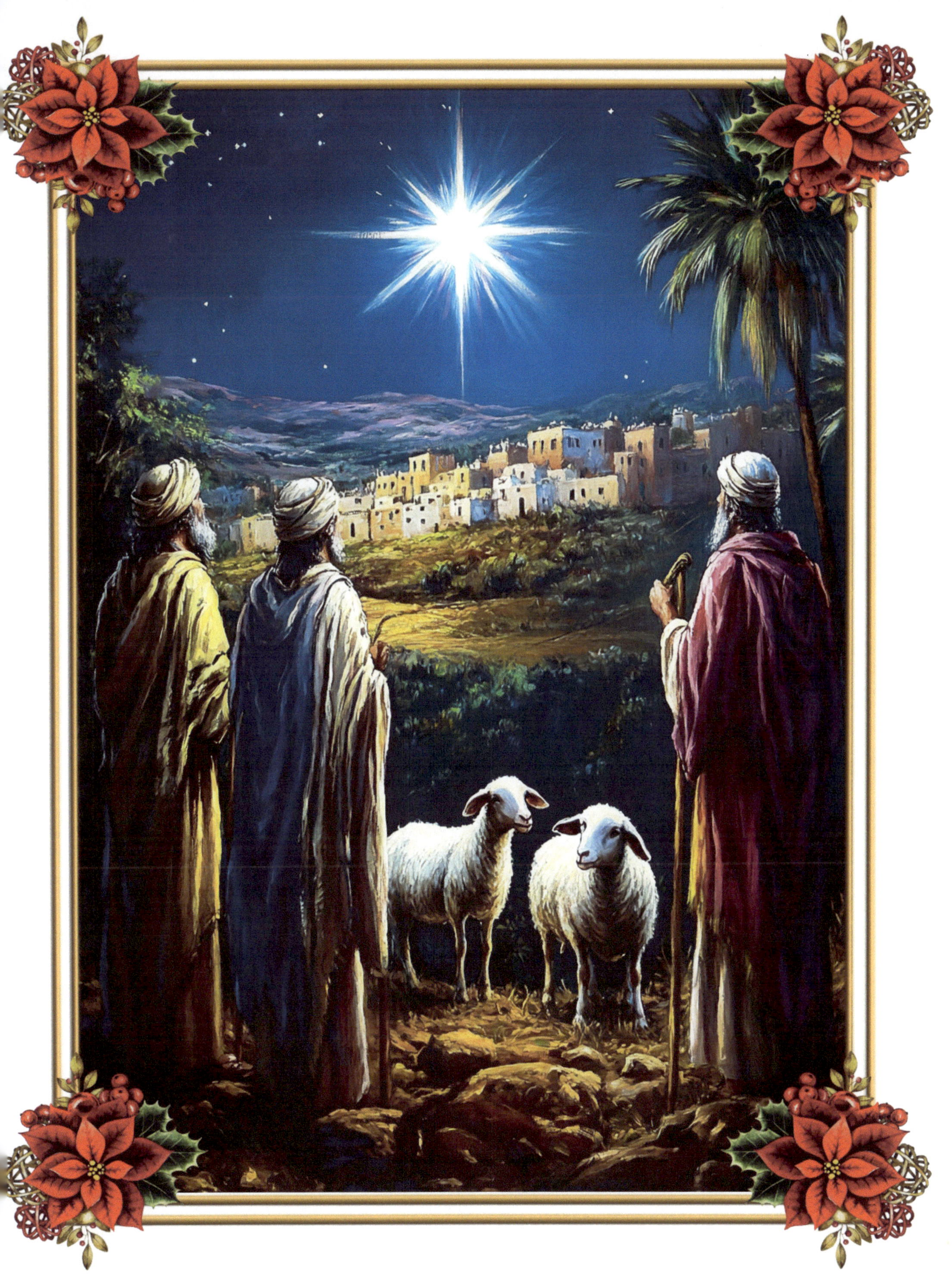

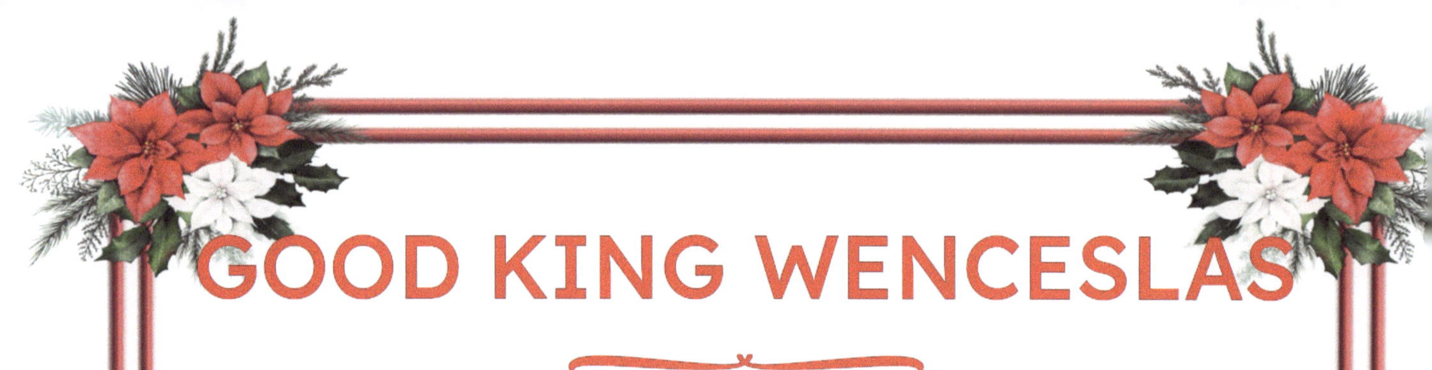

GOOD KING WENCESLAS

Good King Wenceslas looked out
on the Feast of Stephen

When the snow lay round about
deep and crisp and even

Brightly shone the moon that night
tho' the frost was cruel

When a poor man came in sight
gath'ring winter fuel.

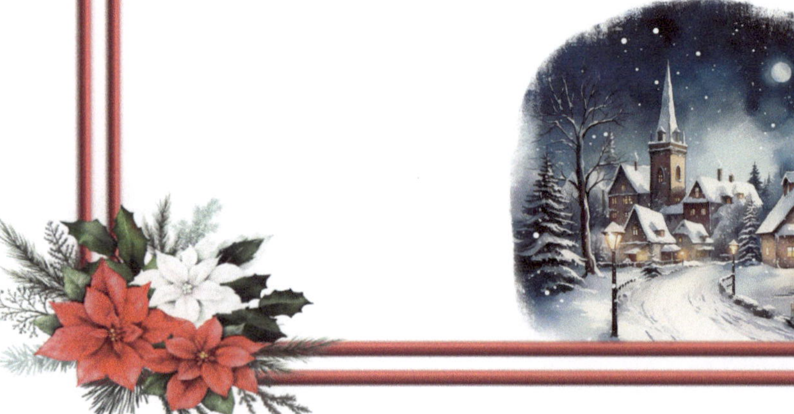

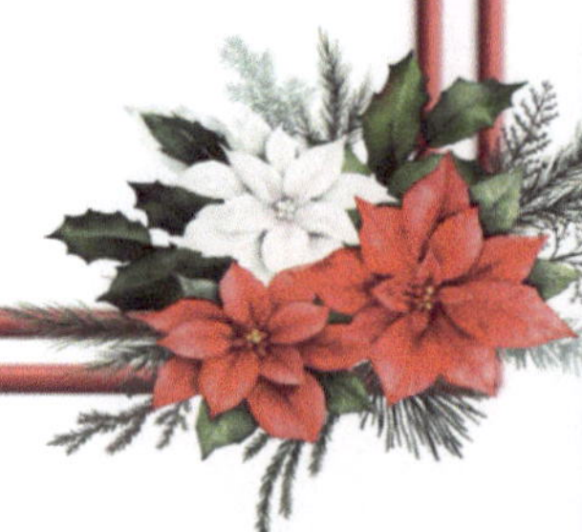

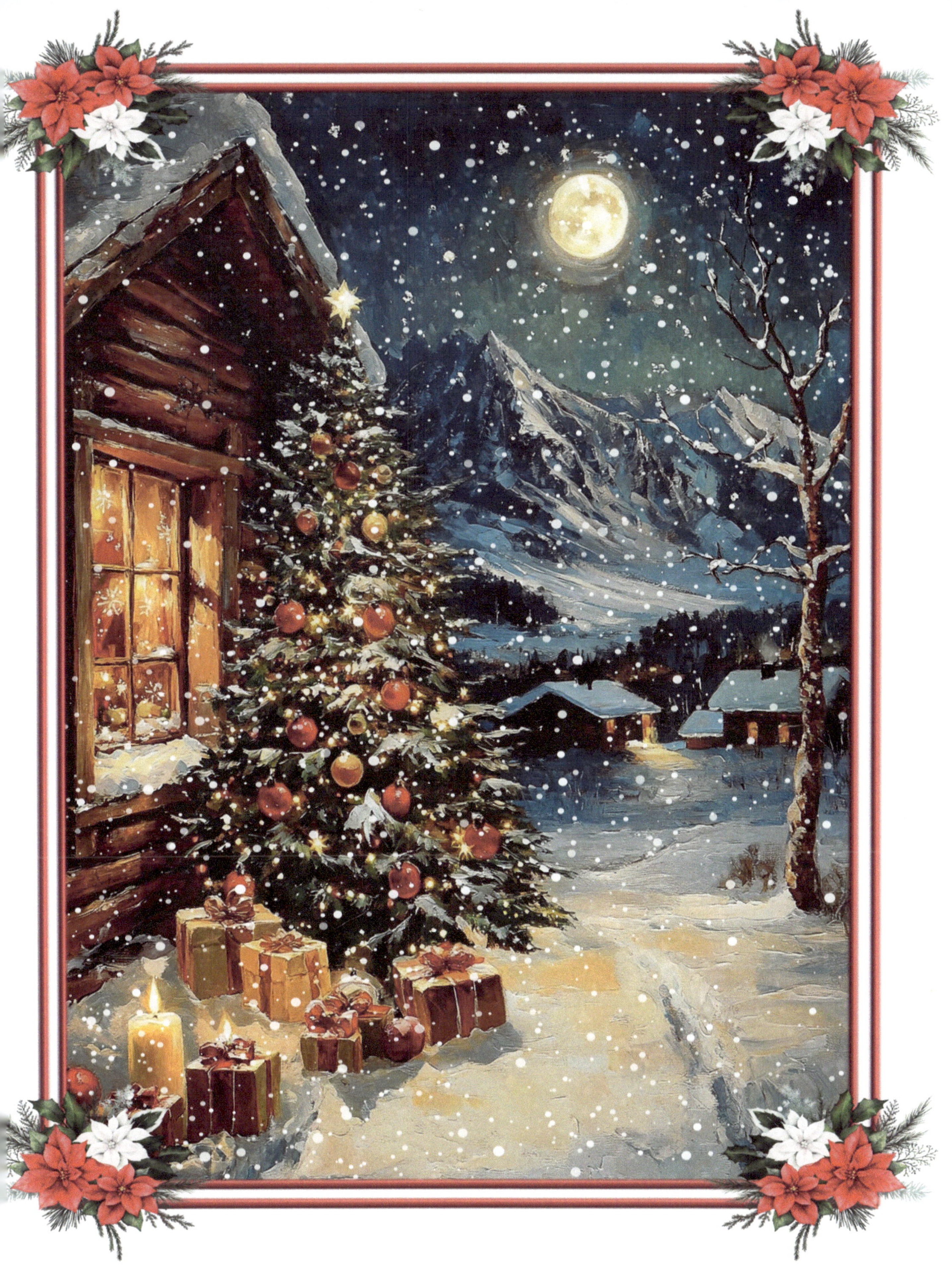

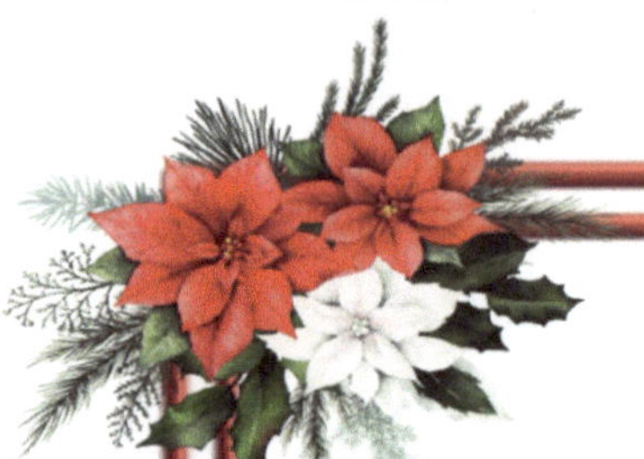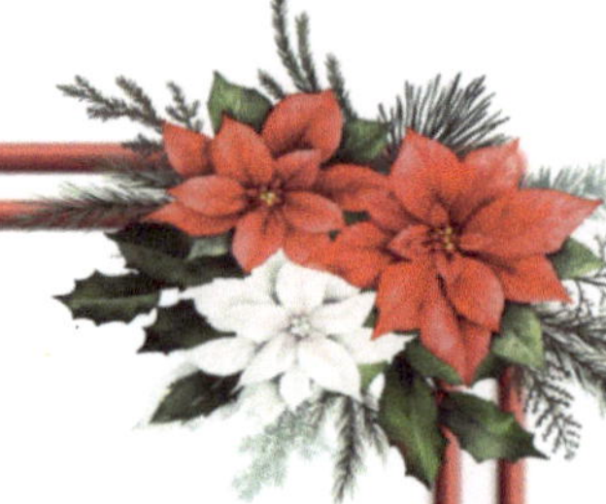

SILVER BELLS

City sidewalks, busy sidewalks
Dressed in holiday style
In the air there's a
feeling of Christmas

Children laughing, people passing
Meeting smile after smile
and on every street corner
you'll hear

Silver bells, silver bells
It's Christmas time in the city
Ring-a-ling, hear them ring
Soon it will be Christmas day

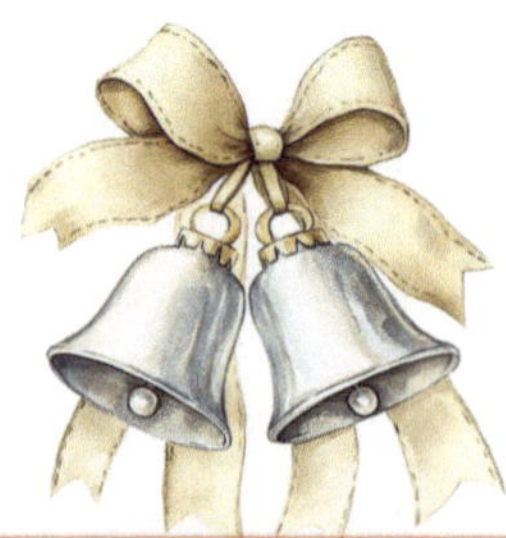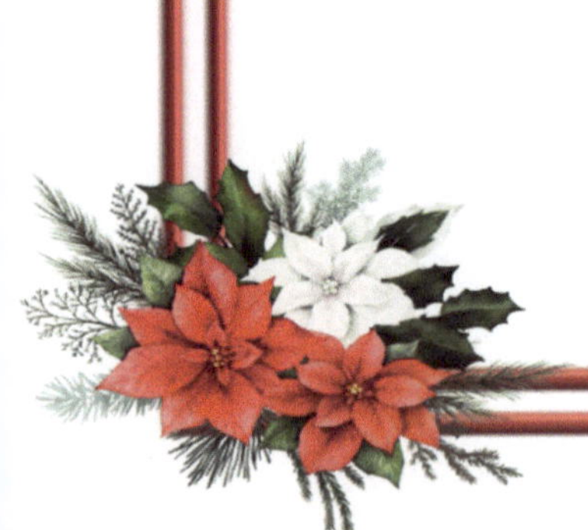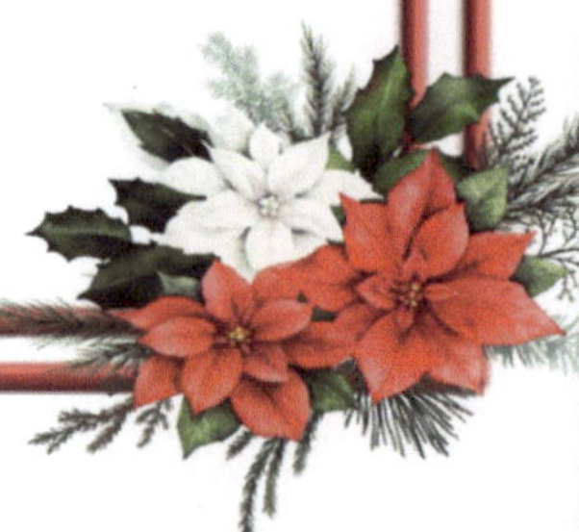

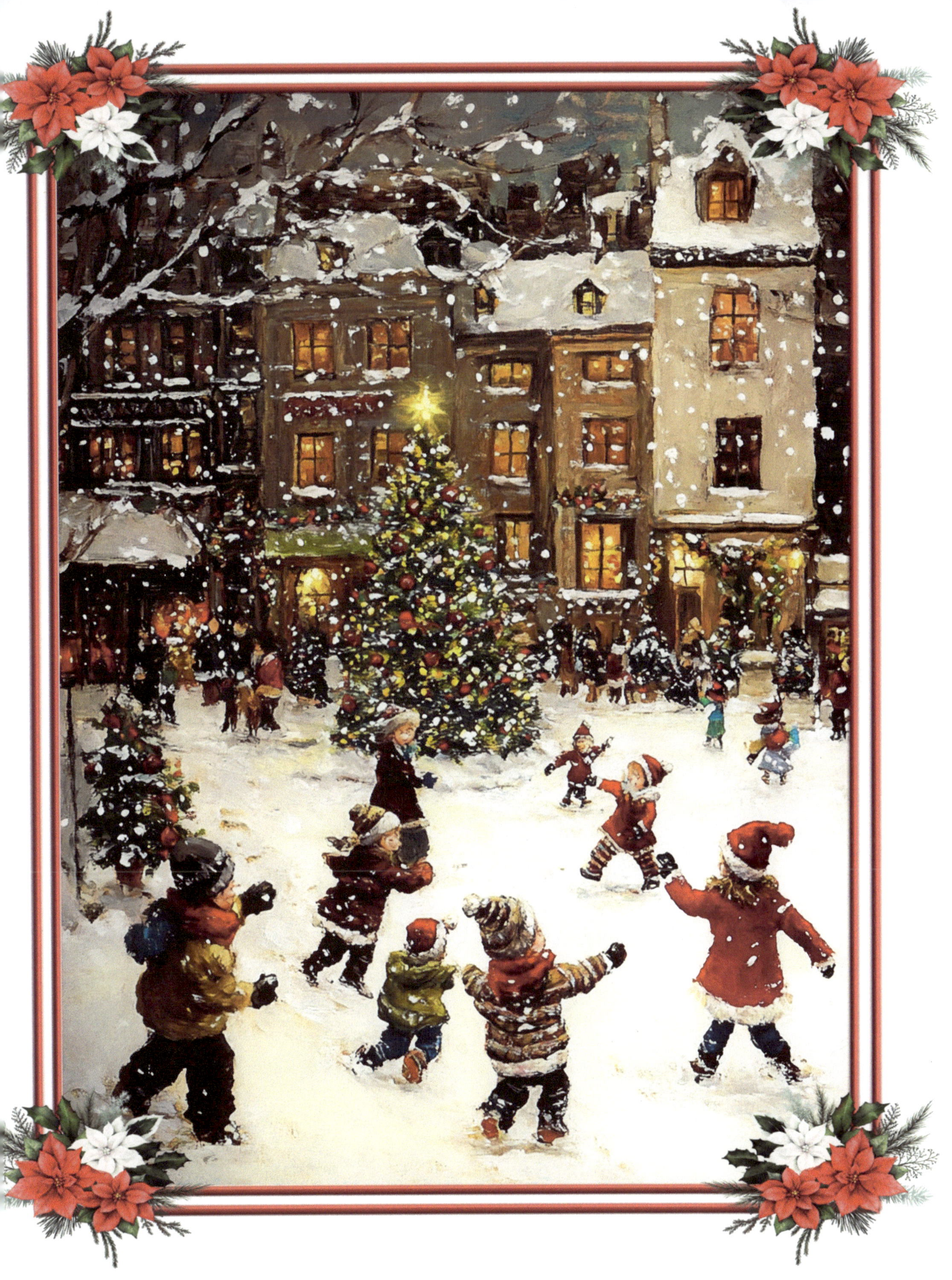

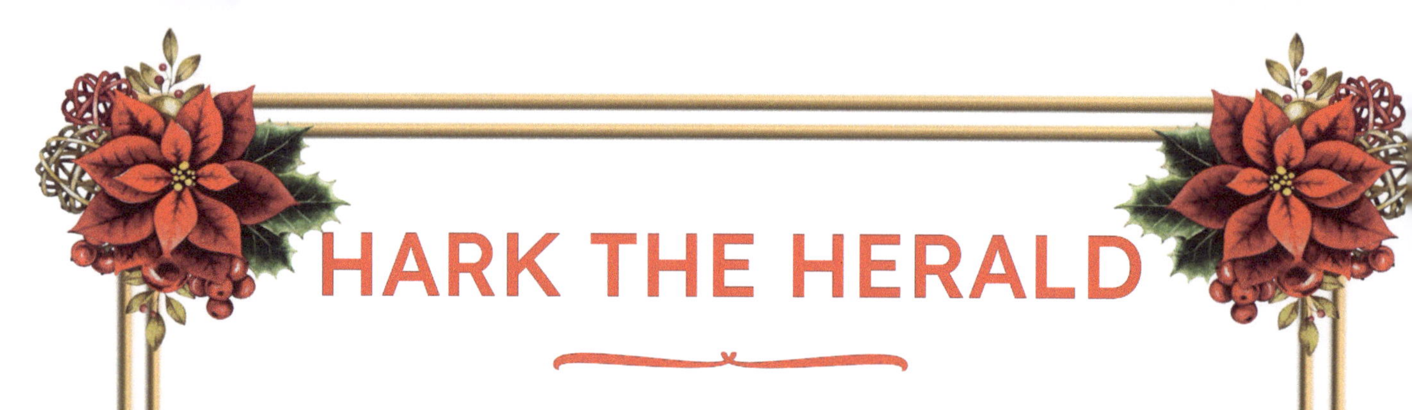

HARK THE HERALD

Hark! the herald angels sing
"Glory to the new born King
peace on earth, and mercy mild
God and sinners reconciled!

Joyful, all ye nations rise
join the triumph of the skies;
with the angelic host proclaim
Christ is born in Bethlehem!

Hark! the herald angels sing
Glory to the new born King!

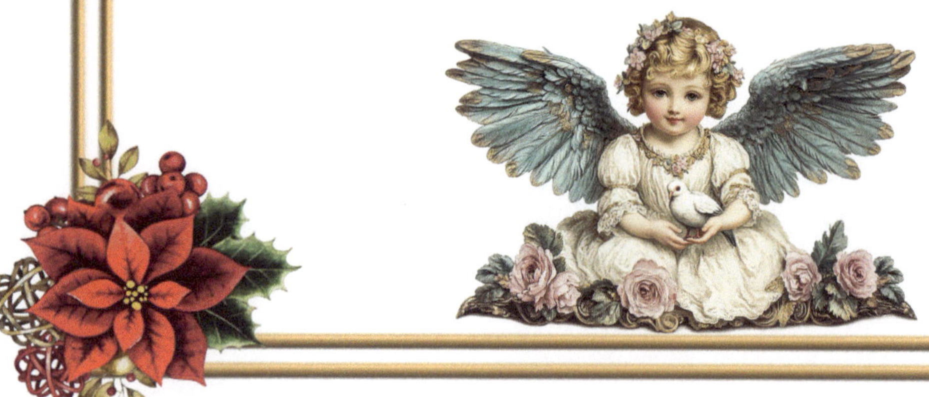

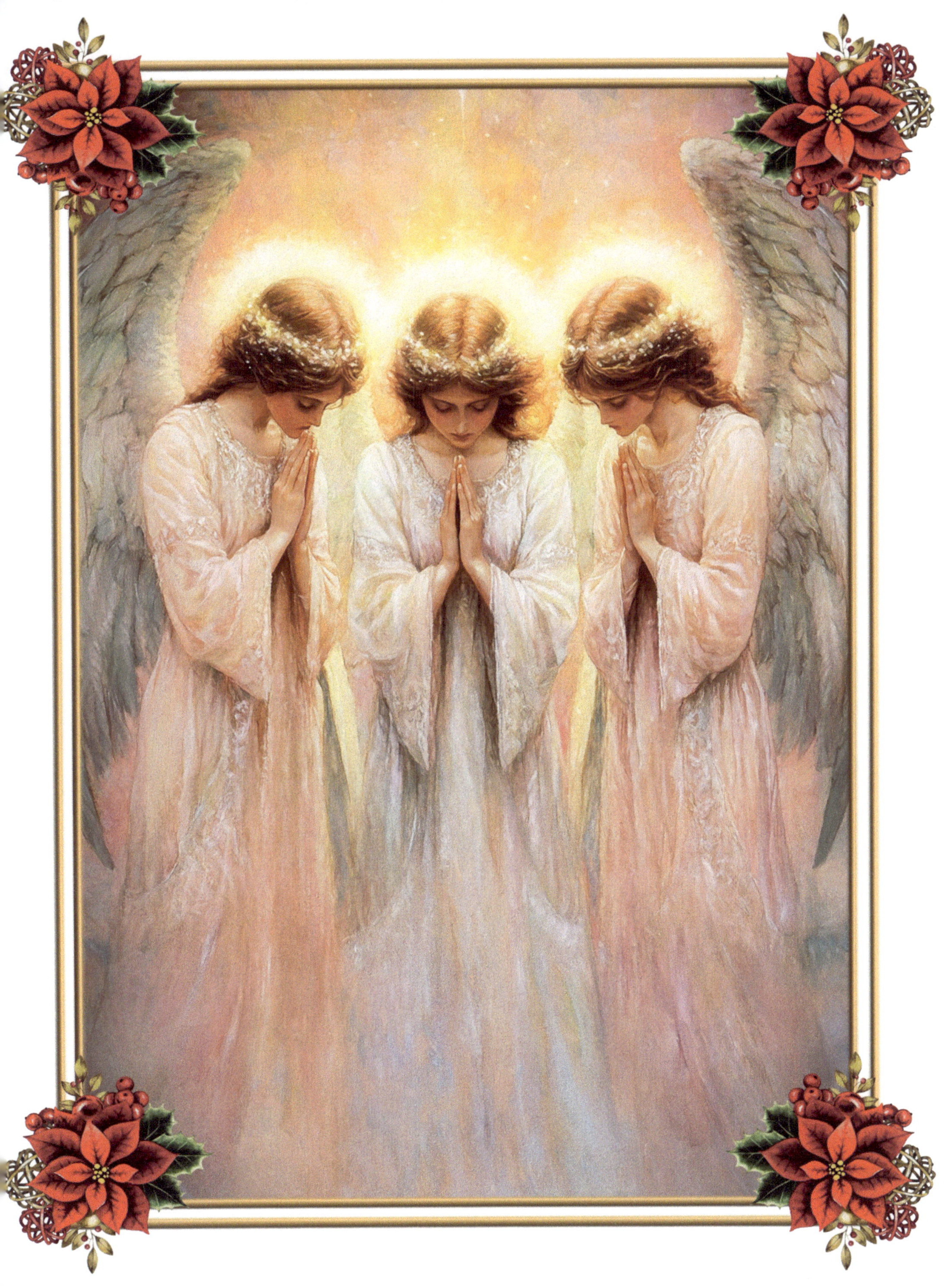

THE HOLLY & THE IVY

The holly and the ivy
now both are full well grown

Of all the trees that are in the wood
the holly bears the crown.

Oh, the rising of the sun
and the running of the deer

The playing of the merry organ,
sweet singing in the choir.

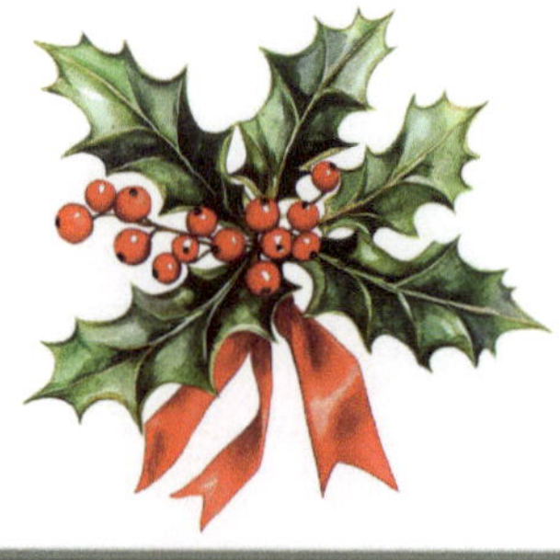

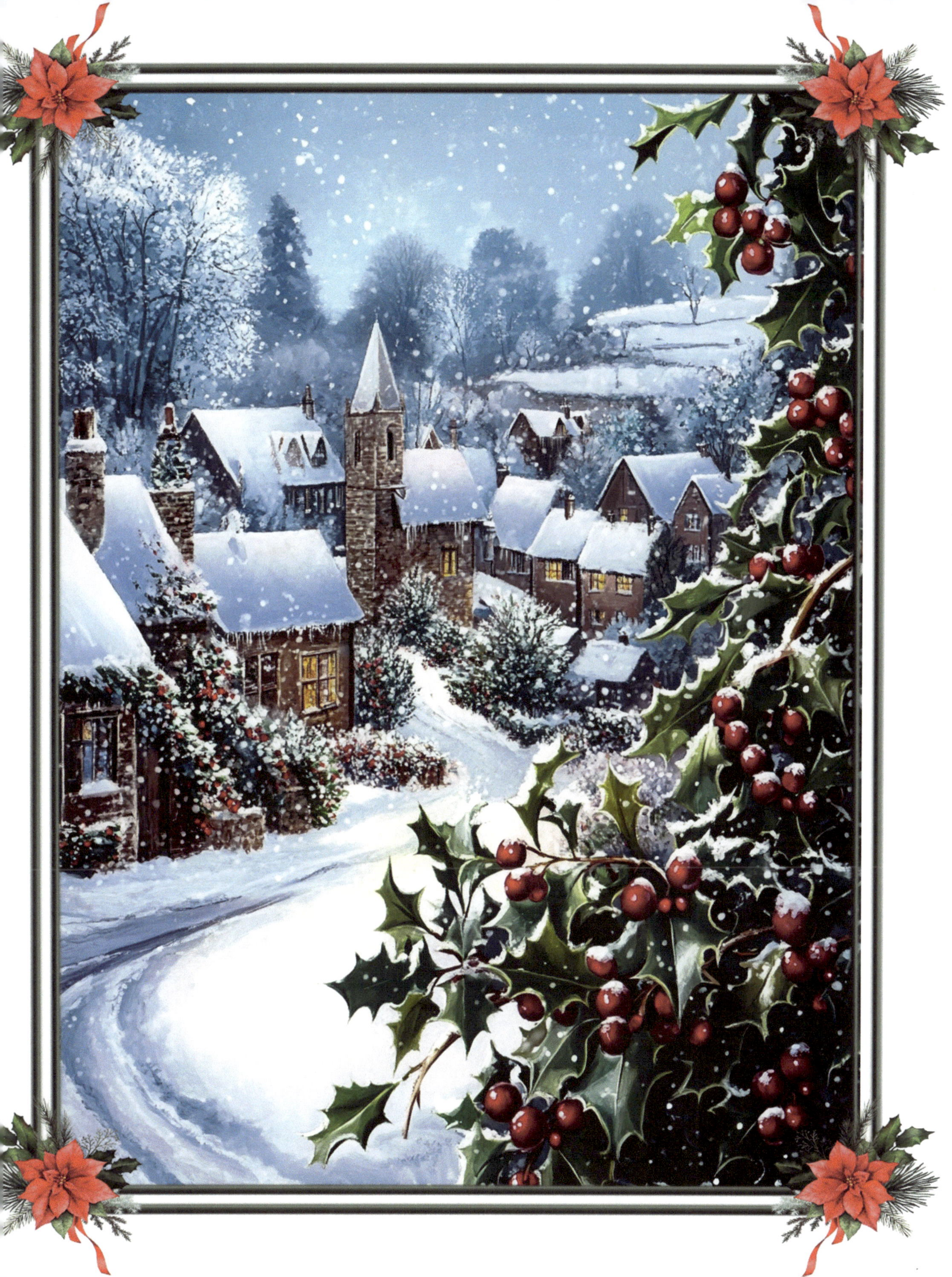

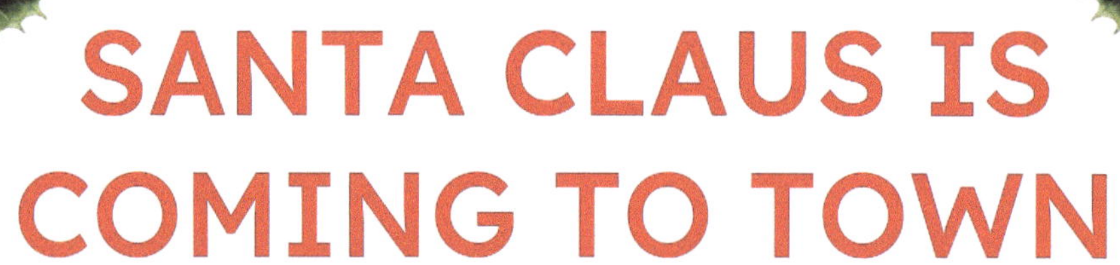

SANTA CLAUS IS COMING TO TOWN

You better watch out
You better not cry

You better not pout
I'm telling you why
Santa Claus is coming to town.

He's making a list
Checking it twice

Gonna find out who's naughty or nice.
Santa Claus is coming to town.

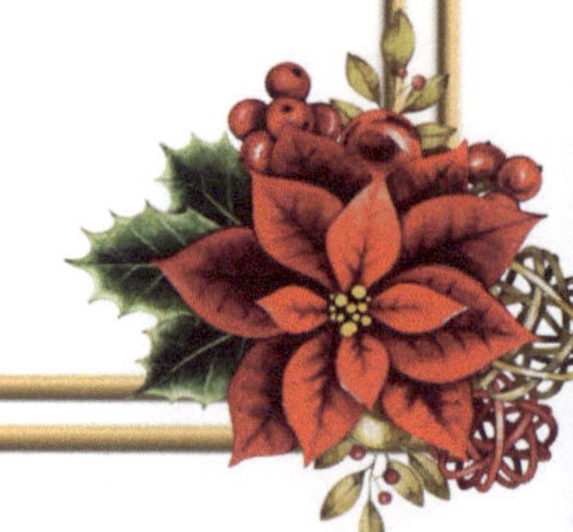

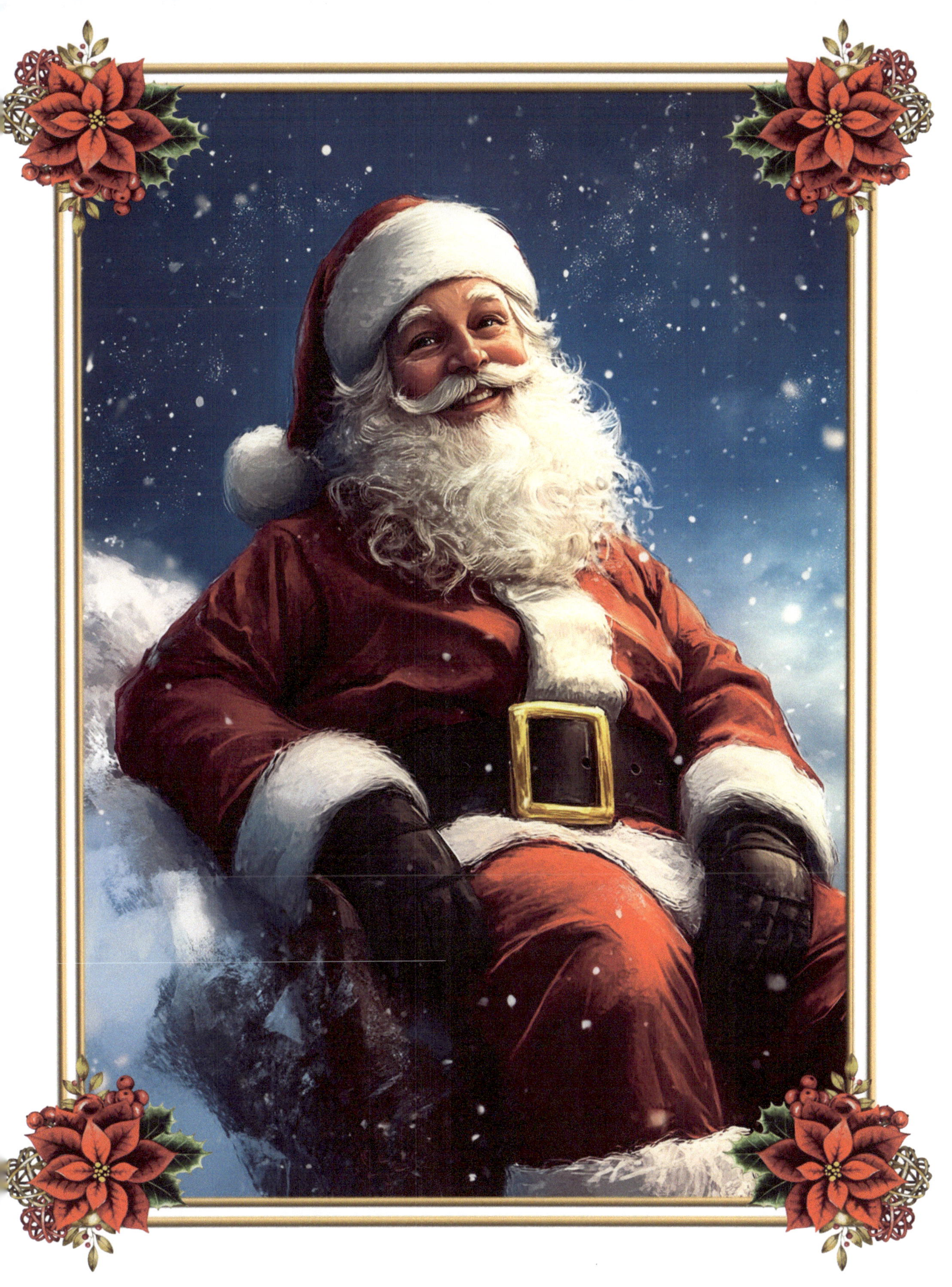

O COME ALL YE FAITHFUL

O come, all ye faithful
Joyful and triumphant!

O come ye, O come ye to Bethlehem;

Come and behold him
Born the King of Angels

O come, let us adore Him
O come, let us adore Him

O come, let us adore Him
Christ the Lord.

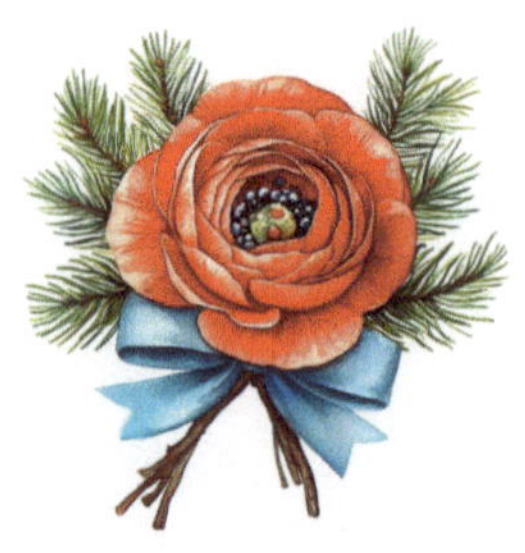

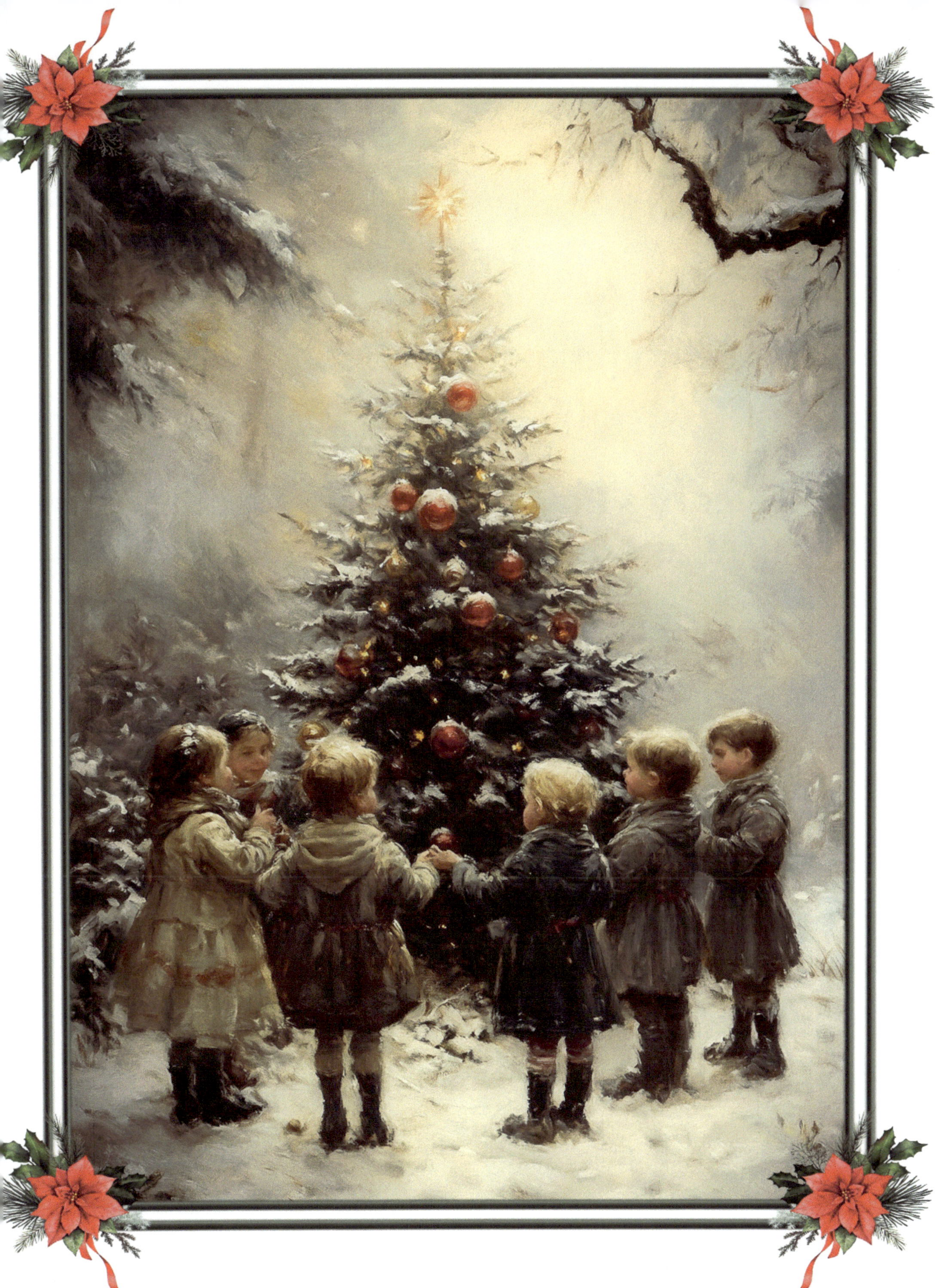

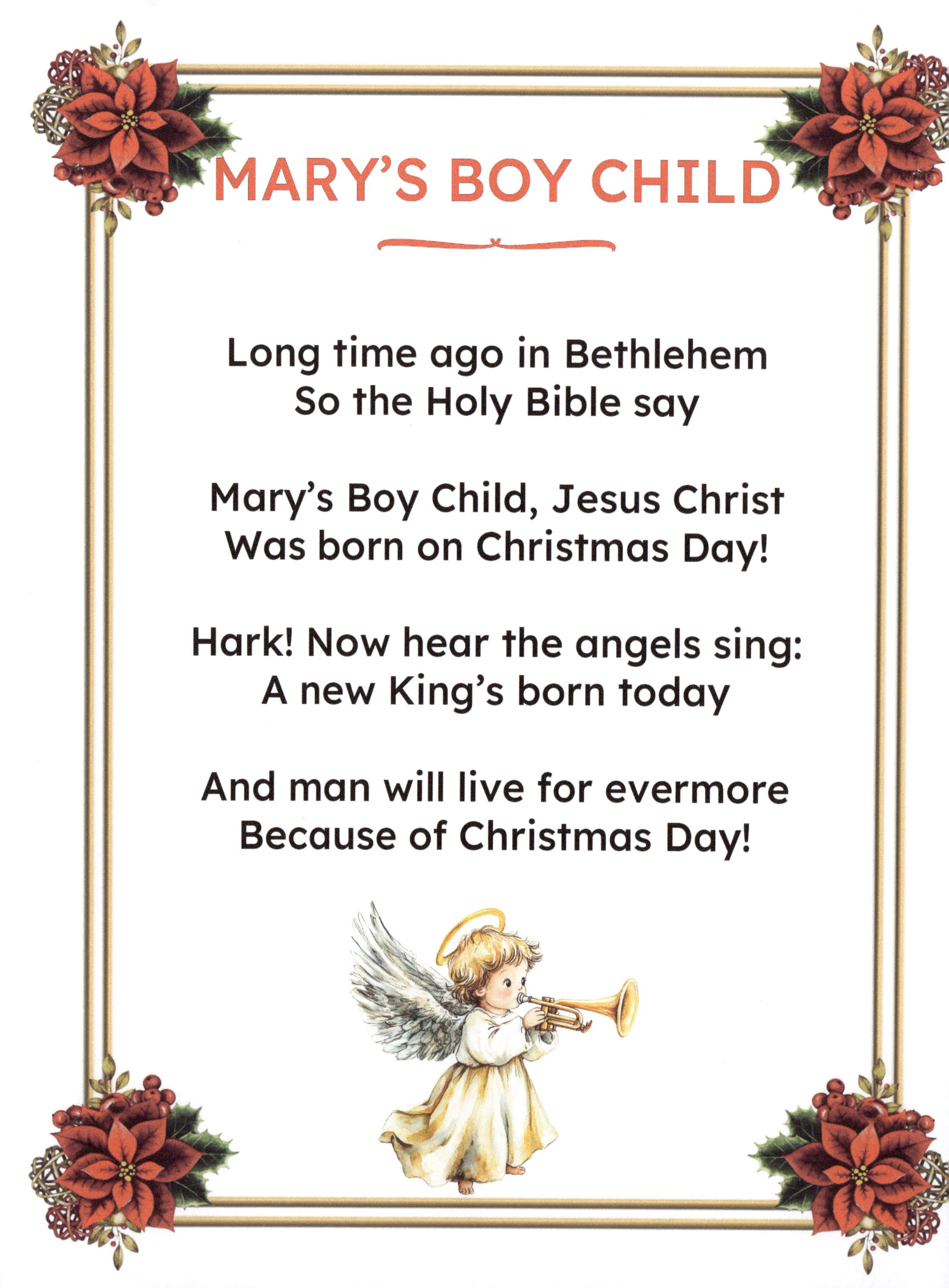
MARY'S BOY CHILD

Long time ago in Bethlehem
So the Holy Bible say

Mary's Boy Child, Jesus Christ
Was born on Christmas Day!

Hark! Now hear the angels sing:
A new King's born today

And man will live for evermore
Because of Christmas Day!

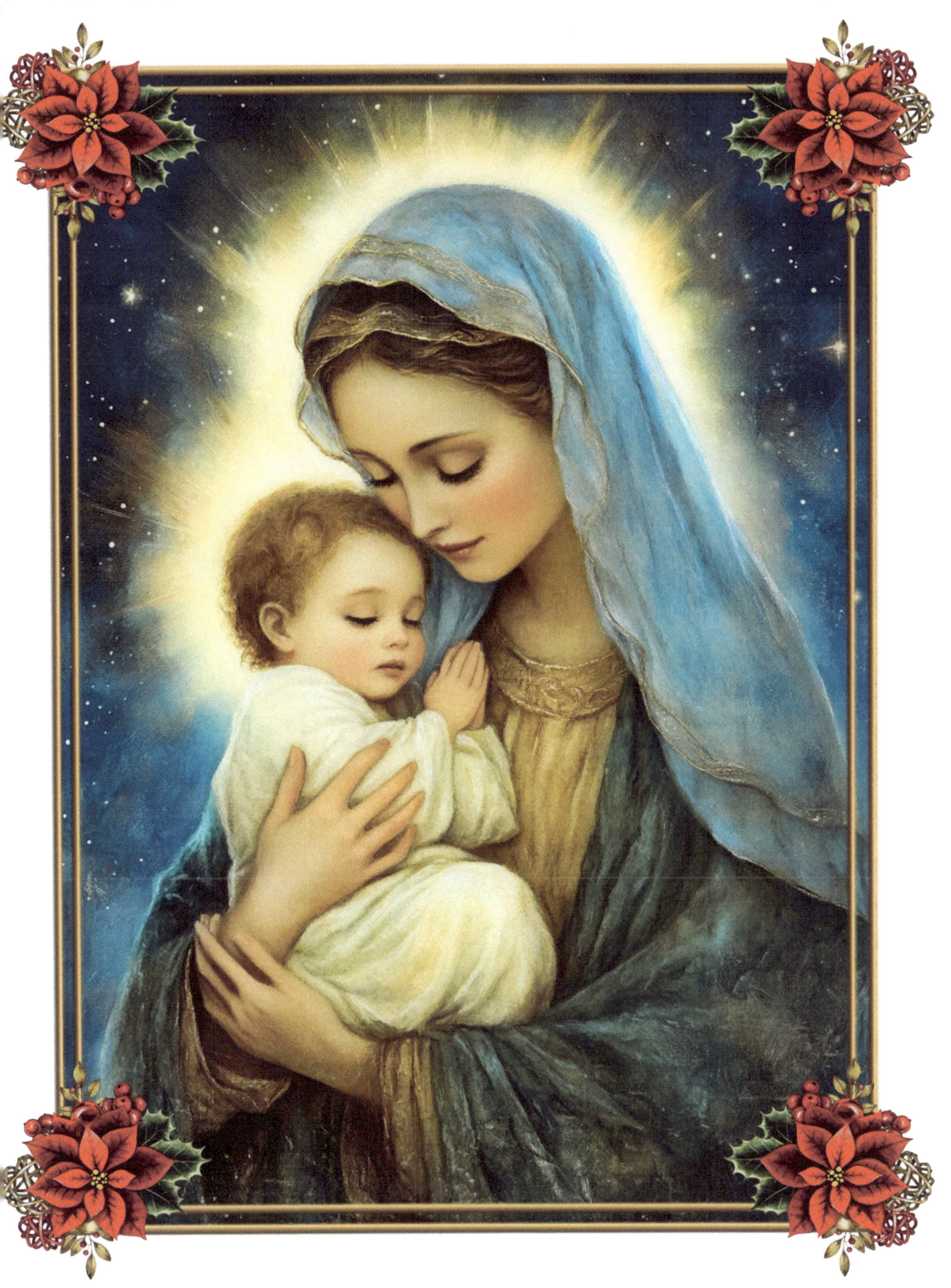

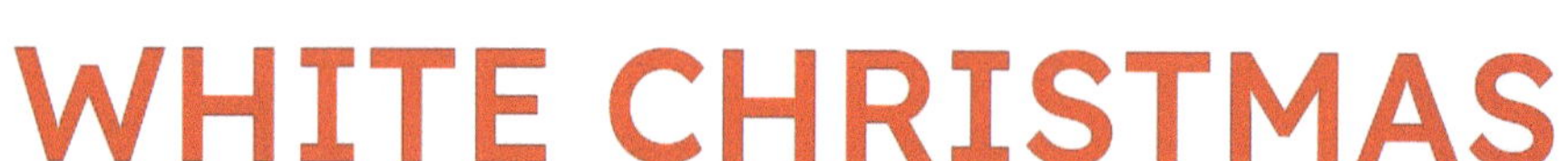

WHITE CHRISTMAS

I'm dreaming of a white Christmas
Just like the ones I used to know
Where the treetops glisten,
and children listen
To hear sleigh bells in the snow.

I'm dreaming of a white Christmas
With every Christmas card I write
May your days be merry and bright
And may all your
Christmases be white.

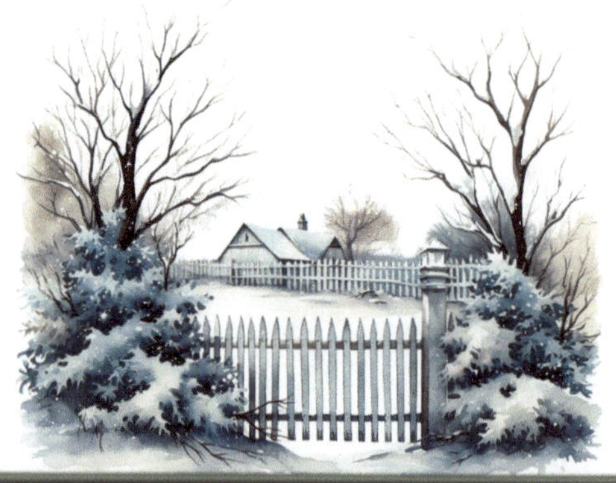

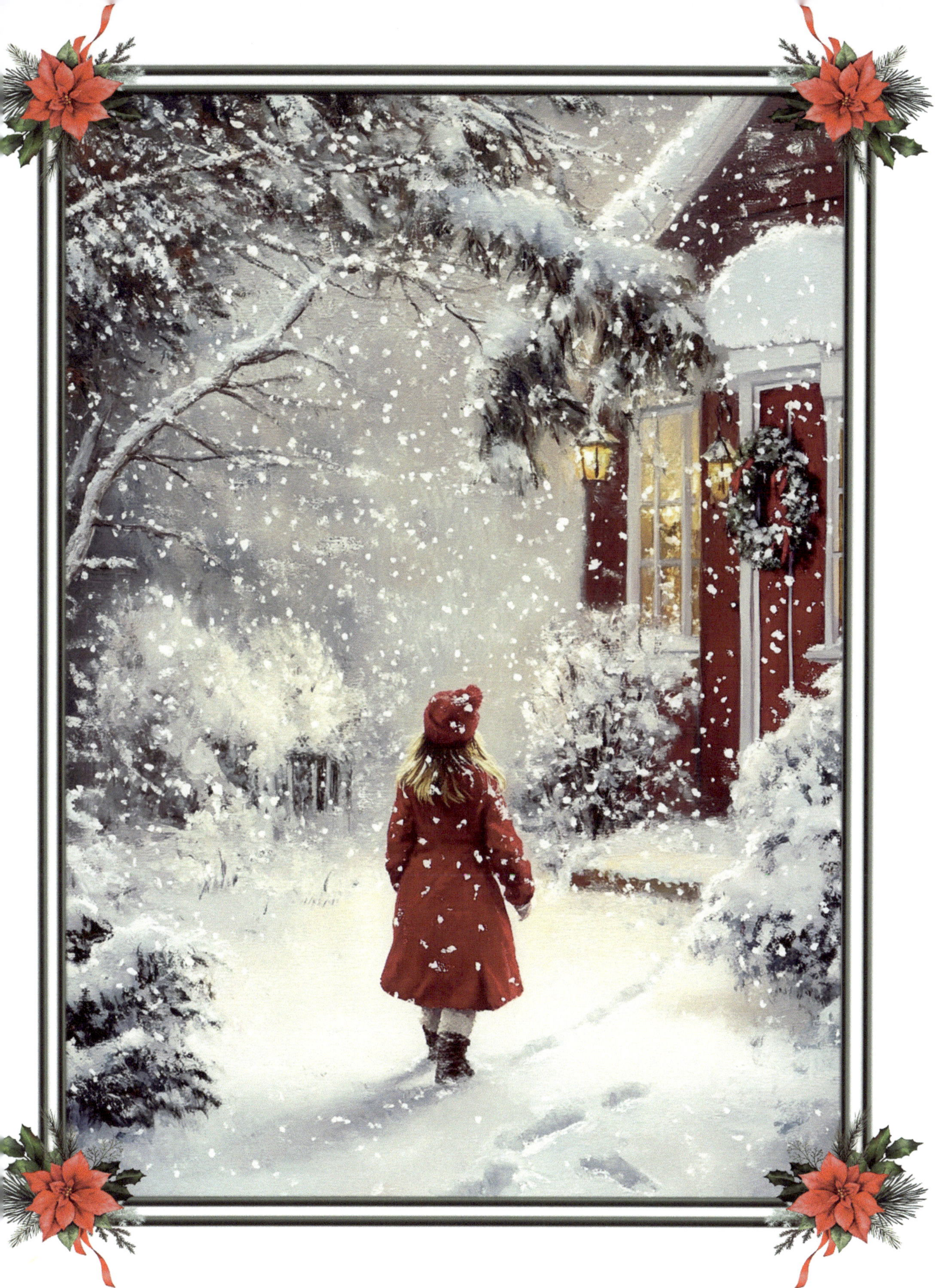

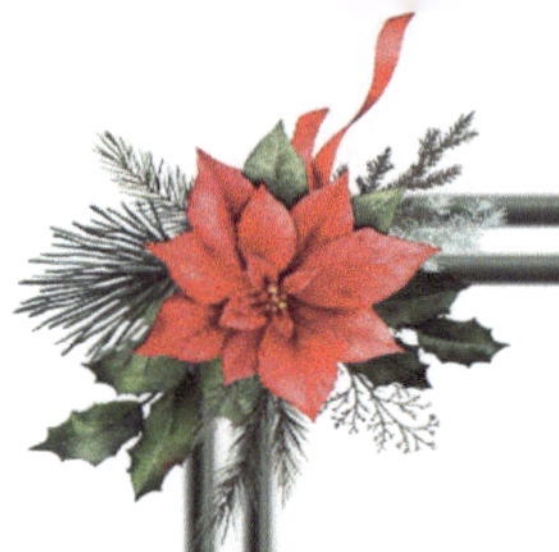
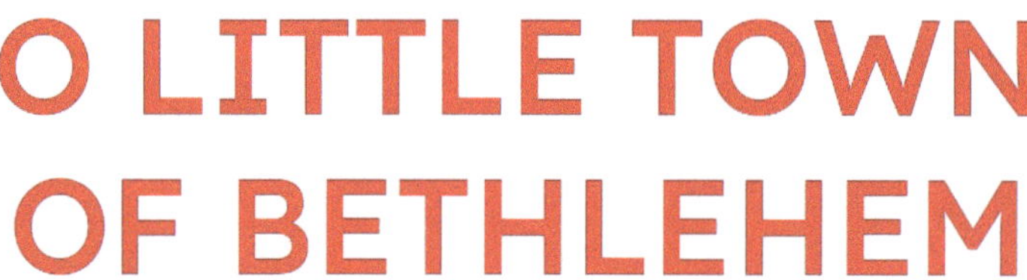

O LITTLE TOWN OF BETHLEHEM

O little town of Bethlehem
How still we see thee lie

Above thy deep and dreamless sleep
The silent stars go by

Yet in thy dark streets shineth
The everlasting Light

The hopes and fears of all the years
Are met in thee tonight

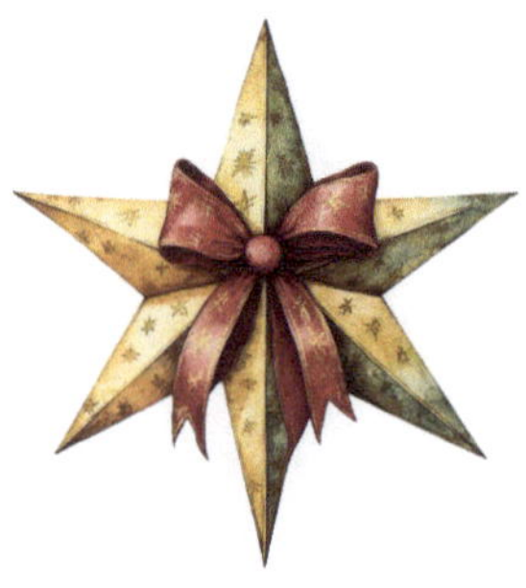

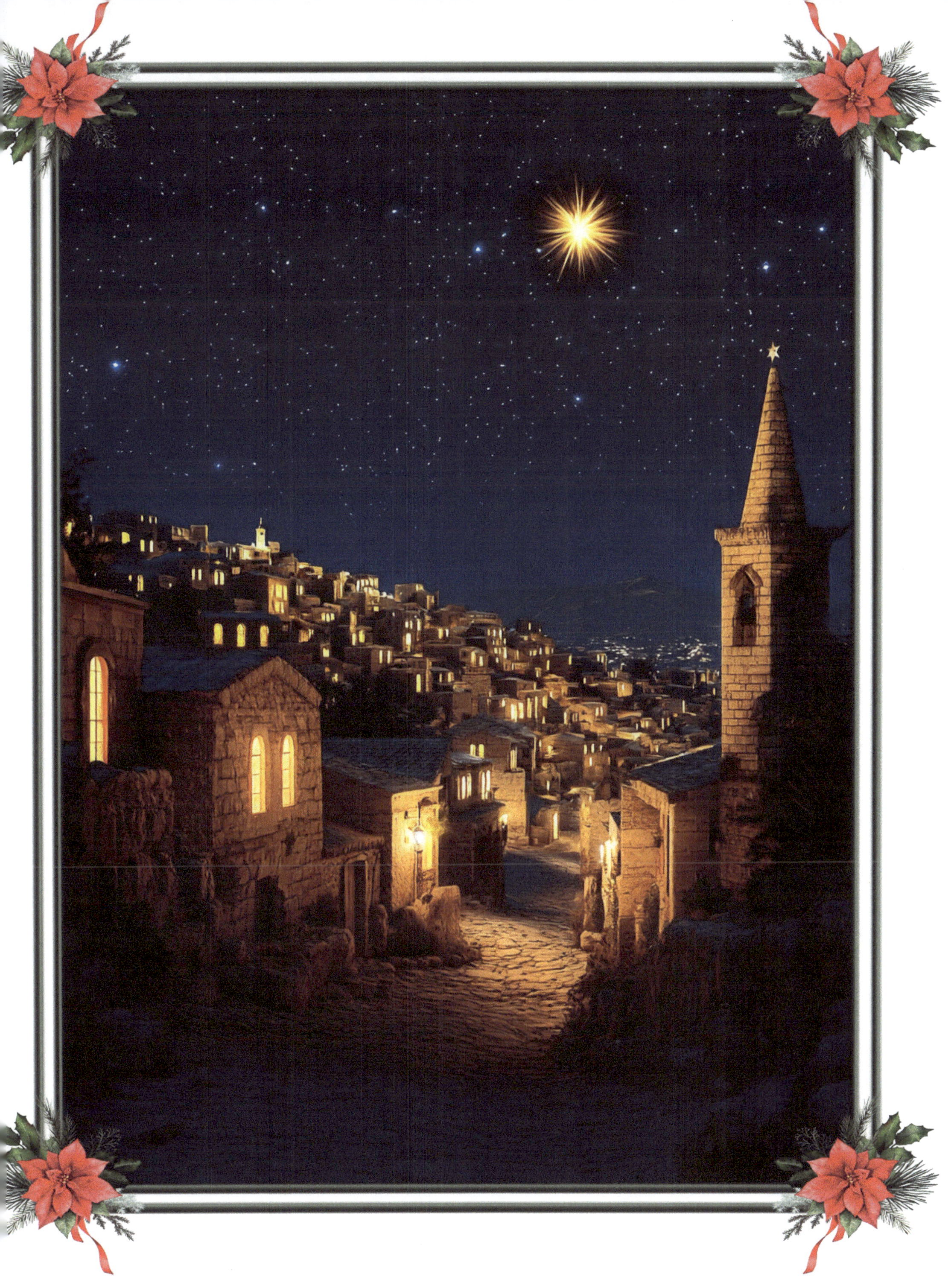

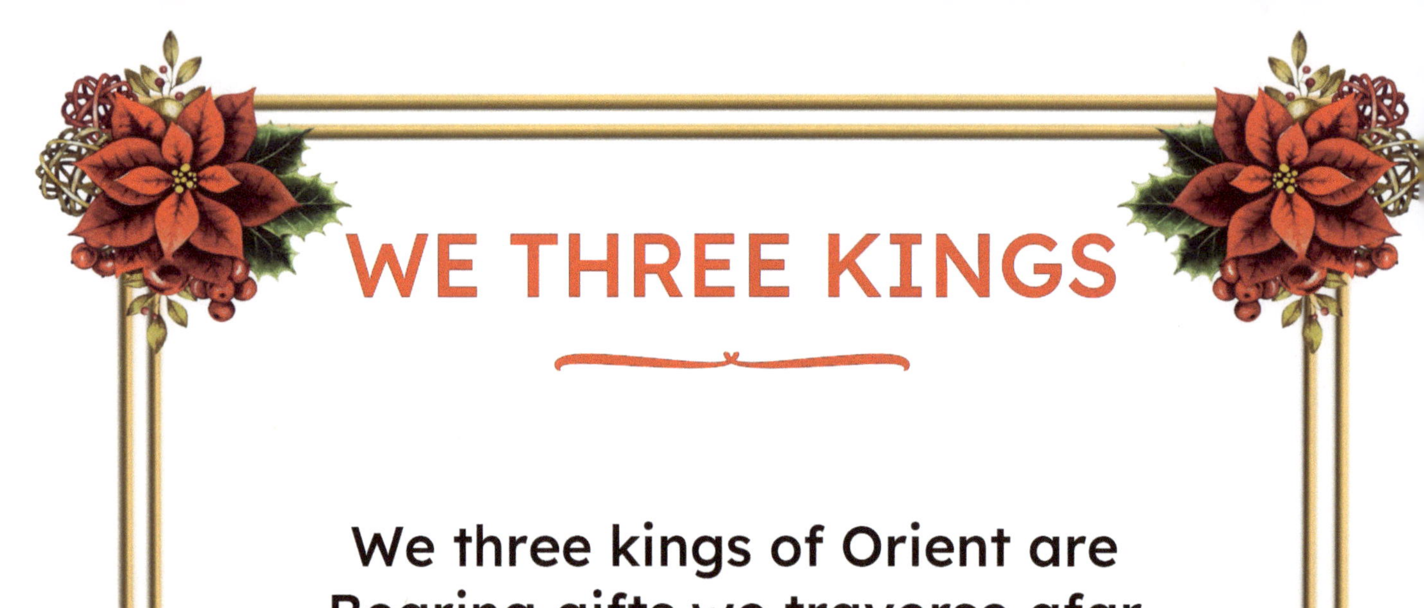

WE THREE KINGS

We three kings of Orient are
Bearing gifts we traverse afar

Field and fountain, moor and mountain
Following yonder star.

O Star of wonder, star of night
Star with royal beauty bright

Westward leading, still proceeding
Guide us to thy Perfect Light.

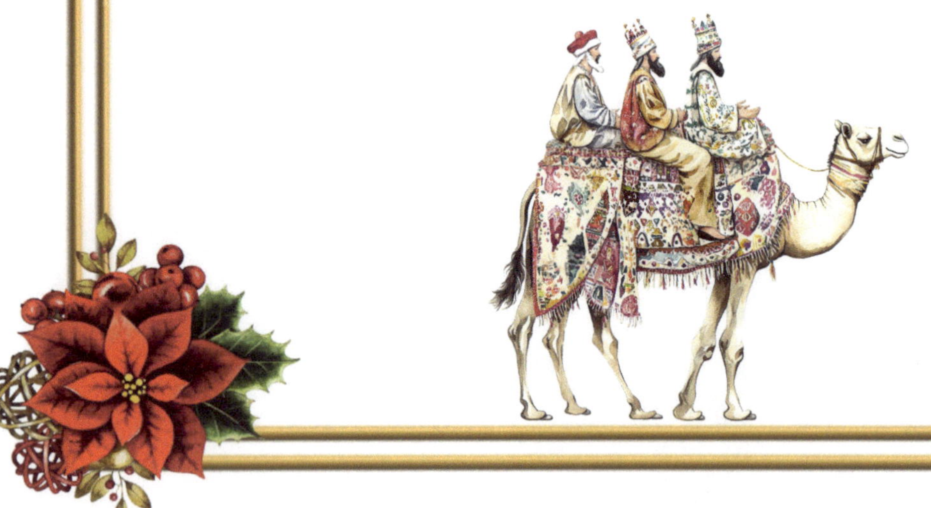

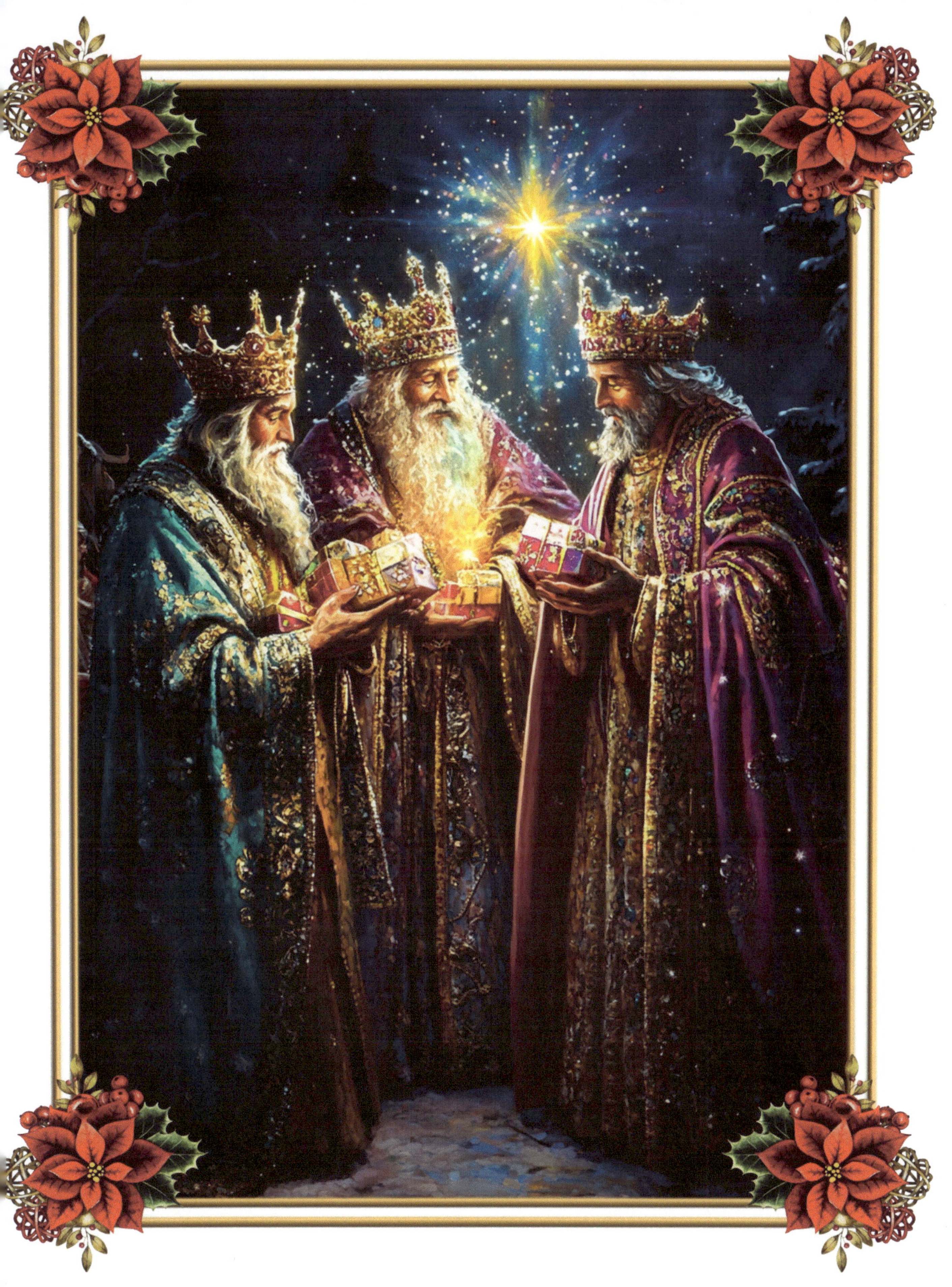

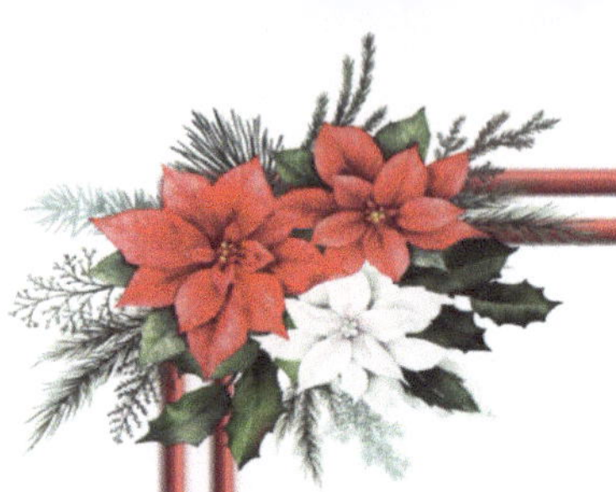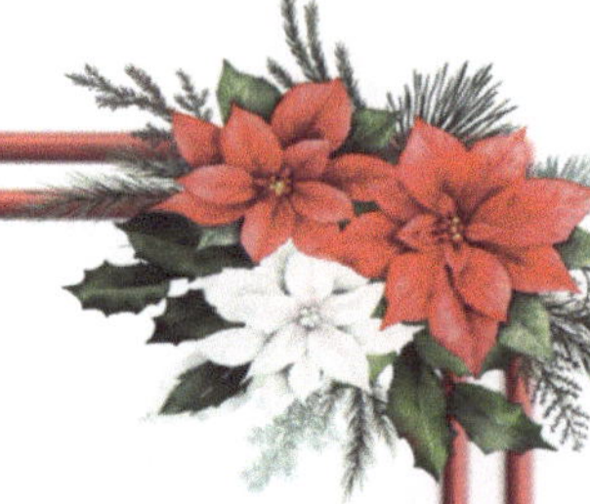

SLEIGH RIDE

Just hear those sleigh bells jingling
ring ting tingling too

Come on, it's lovely weather
for a sleigh ride together with you

Outside the snow is falling
and friends are calling "Yoo hoo,"

Come on, it's lovely weather
for a sleigh ride together with you.

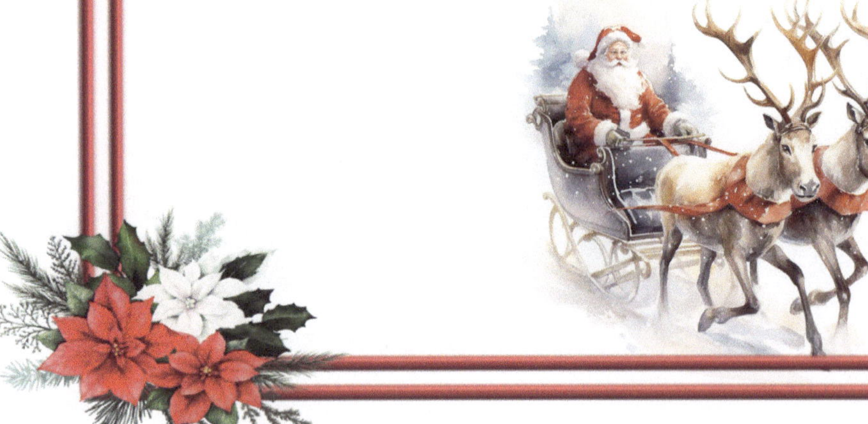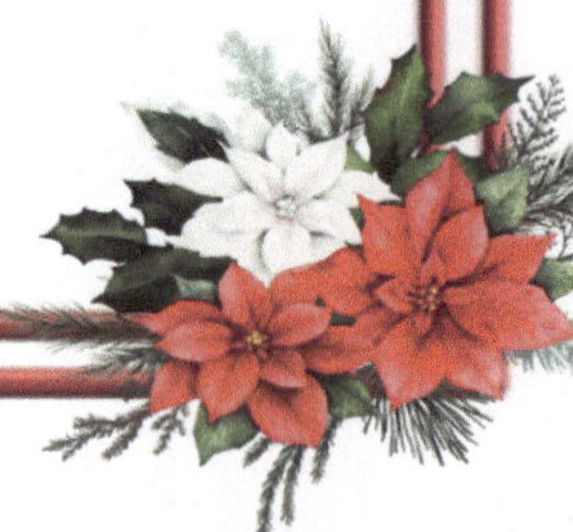

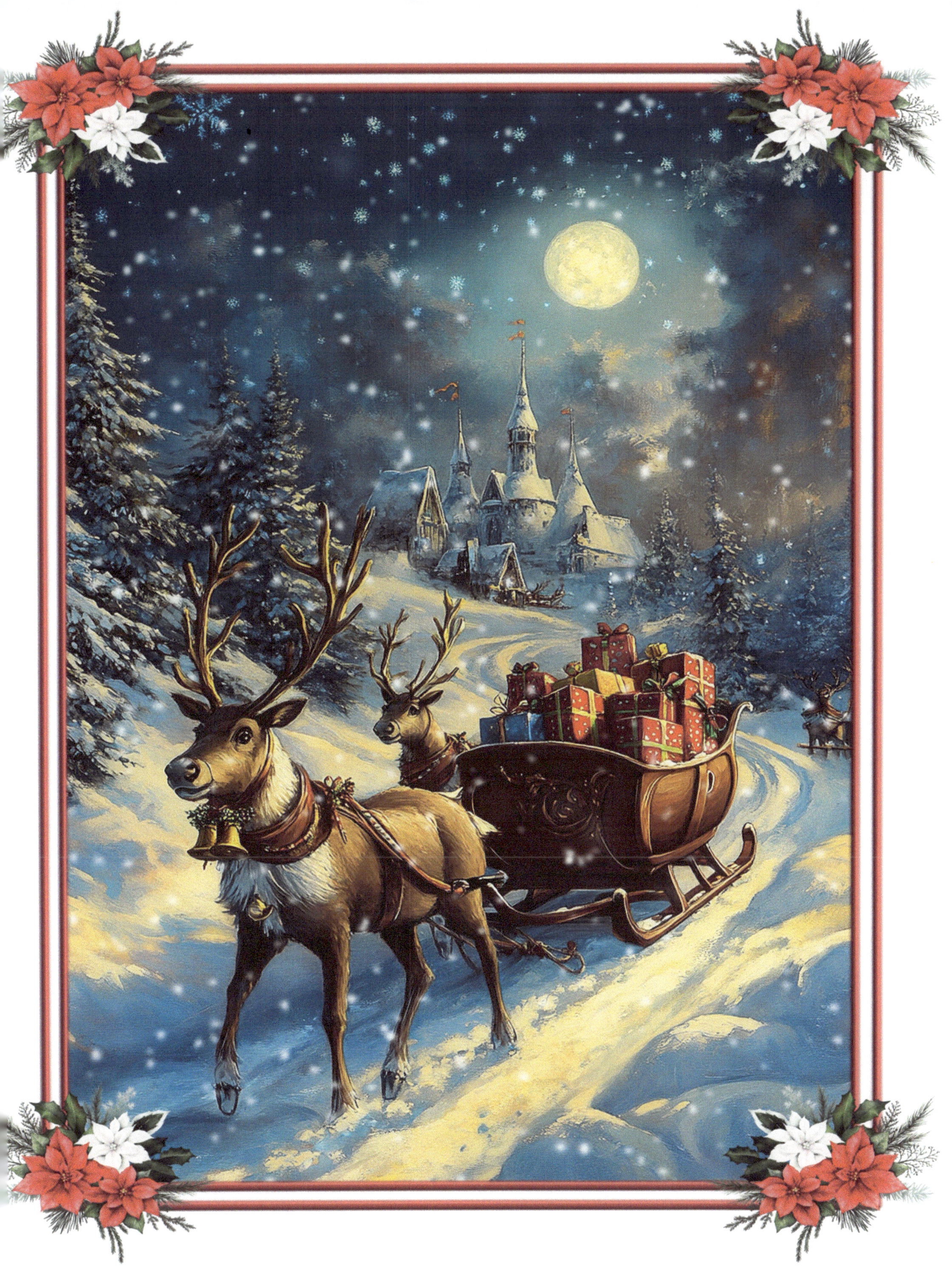

WE WISH YOU A MERRY CHRISTMAS

We wish you a Merry Christmas
We wish you a Merry Christmas

We wish you a Merry Christmas
and a Happy New Year.

Good tidings we bring
to you and your kin.

We wish you a Merry Christmas
and a Happy New Year.

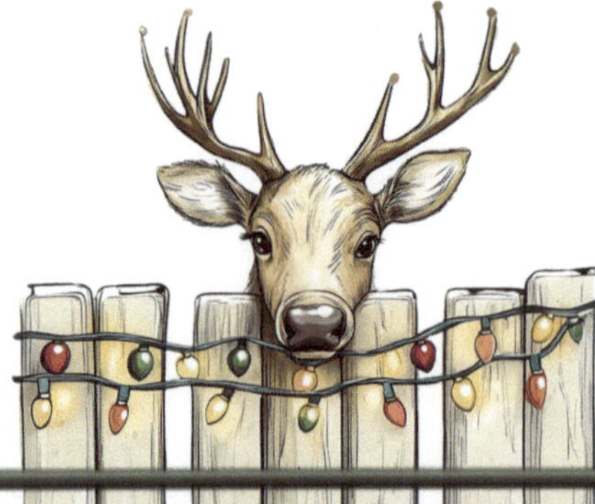

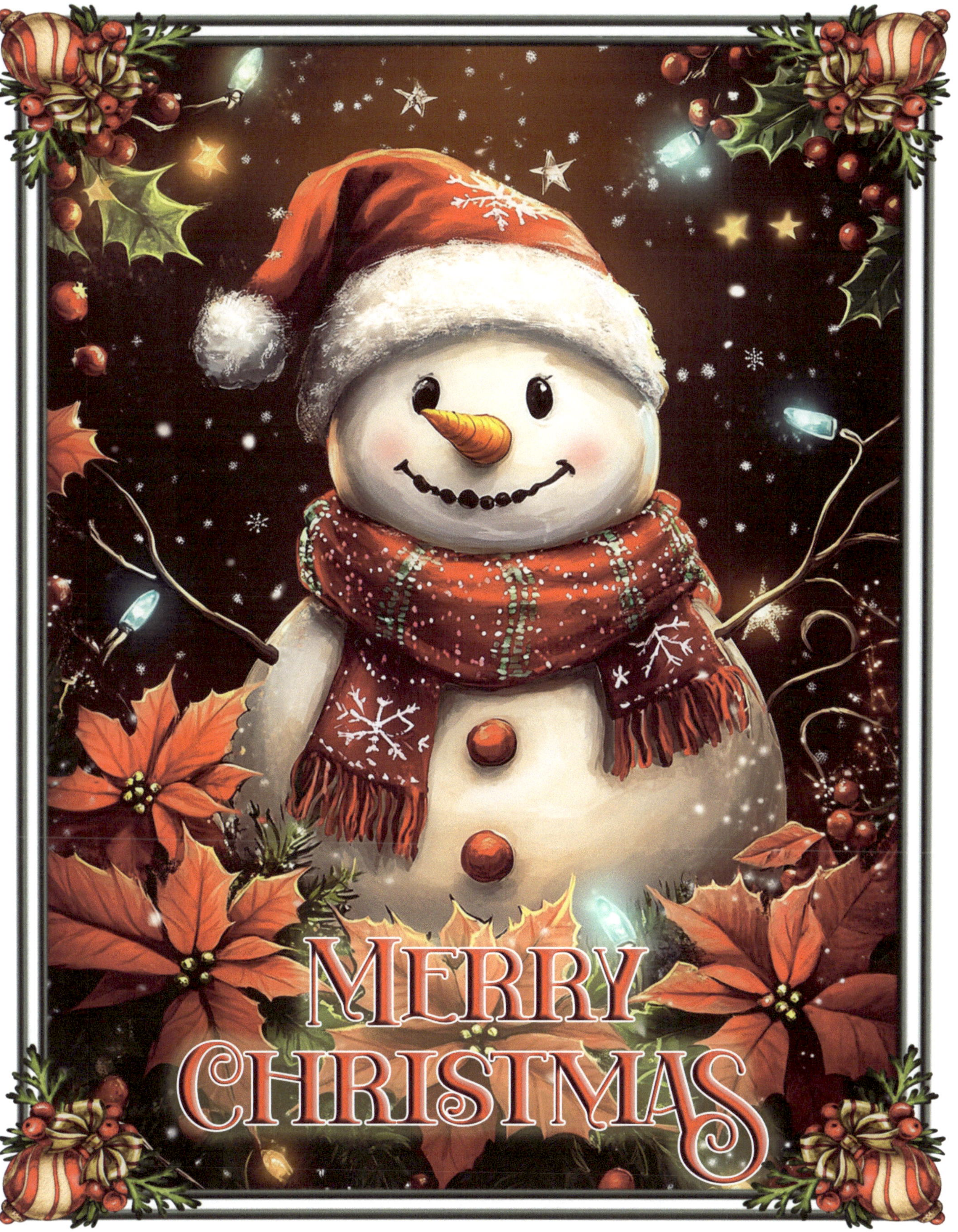

MERRY CHRISTMAS